TABLE OF CONTENTS

M000305084

76896

Top 20 Test Taking Tips

1. Carefully follow all the test registration procedures
2. Know the test directions, duration, topics, question types, how many questions
3. Setup a flexible study schedule at least 3-4 weeks before test day
4. Study during the time of day you are most alert, relaxed, and stress free
5. Maximize your learning style; visual learner use visual study aids, auditory learner use auditory study aids
6. Focus on your weakest knowledge base
7. Find a study partner to review with and help clarify questions
8. Practice, practice, practice
9. Get a good night's sleep; don't try to cram the night before the test
10. Eat a well balanced meal
11. Know the exact physical location of the testing site; drive the route to the site prior to test day
12. Bring a set of ear plugs; the testing center could be noisy
13. Wear comfortable, loose fitting, layered clothing to the testing center; prepare for it to be either cold or hot during the test
14. Bring at least 2 current forms of ID to the testing center
15. Arrive to the test early; be prepared to wait and be patient
16. Eliminate the obviously wrong answer choices, then guess the first remaining choice
17. Pace yourself; don't rush, but keep working and move on if you get stuck
18. Maintain a positive attitude even if the test is going poorly
19. Keep your first answer unless you are positive it is wrong
20. Check your work, don't make a careless mistake

Exam Overview

Every nursing program is different, and you may or may not be tested on all of the following sections:

- Math: 50-item exam. Focuses on math needed for calculation of Drugs and Solutions. 50 minutes.
- Reading Comprehension: 47-item exam. Reading scenarios that are health related. The reading scenarios pop up on the screen. Students can move around the windows to see the entire scenario. 50 minutes
- Vocabulary and General Knowledge: 50-item exam. Contains basic vocabulary that is often used in health care fields. 50 minutes.
- Grammar: 50-item exam. Contains basic grammar. Time allotment: 50 minutes
- Chemistry: 25-item exam. 25 minutes.
- Anatomy and Physiology (A&P): 25-item exam. 25 minutes.
- Biology: 25-item exam. 25 minutes.
- Not Scored Sections:
- Learning Styles: Identifies individual learning style and prints test-taking and study tips best suited for the individual's learning style and relates these recommendations to nursing curricula.
- Personality Style: Uses concepts related to introversion and extroversion to classify the student's personality style. Explanations are printed at the conclusion of the exam to let the student know how to use his/her personality style to be successful in a nursing education program.

English Language

Reading Comprehension

The reading comprehension portion of the exam requires the student to answer questions based on a passage that they have read. These questions are related to comprehension of reading measure the students' ability to comprehend meaning, identify the main idea, finding meaning of words in context, passage comprehension, making logical inferences, etc. There are 47 reading comprehension items, and 50 minutes are allowed for this part of the exam.

Preparing for the test

One of the best techniques for increasing reading comprehension is to read as much and as often as possible. Expand your literary horizons by reading a variety of publications. Read things like fiction stories, medical journals, comic books, and newspapers. This forces your mind to encounter new words and concepts. Keep reading materials in places where you will have idle time, such as the bathroom and your car. When you are waiting in line at the bank or pumping gas, you can thumb through a news magazine or read a chapter of a book. Tuck a book or pamphlet into your purse or pocket and read while standing in line at the grocery store. If you are using the Internet to decide which movie to see, read some reviews for each movie.

Skimming

On standardized tests, the reading comprehension section will generally contain a paragraph followed by a series of questions. Students may find it helpful to read each of the questions before reading the paragraph. This will alert the student to the specific details they should look for while reading. While reading the paragraph, the student will discover that the answers to the questions are more obvious.

When answers do not readily appear in the course of reading, it is useful to reread the question and carefully consider each possible answer choice. Skimming questions before reading a paragraph can also provide a basic idea of the content of the article. For example, if all of the questions deal with pacemakers, the student can expect an article about that topic. Students should also pay attention to the nature of the questions, whether they are general or specific. Questions that ask for names or dates indicate that the student should note these details as they read.

Since your first task when you begin reading is to identify the topic of the selection, begin to read by quickly skimming the passage for the general idea, stopping to read only the first sentence of each paragraph. A paragraph's first sentence is usually the main topic sentence, and it gives you a summary of the content of the paragraph.

This will give you a general idea about what it is about, as well as what is the expected topic in each paragraph.

Key words

Each question will contain clues as to where to find the answer in the passage. Do not just randomly search through the passage for the correct answer to each question. Search scientifically. Find key word(s) or ideas in the question that are going to either contain or be near the correct answer. These are typically nouns, verbs, numbers, or phrases in the question that will probably be duplicated in the passage. Once you have identified those key word(s) or idea, skim the passage quickly to find where those key word(s) or idea appears. The correct answer choice will be nearby.
Example:

> What caused Martin to suddenly return to Paris?

The key word is Paris. Skim the passage quickly to find where this word appears. The answer will be close by that word.

However, sometimes key words in the question are not repeated in the passage. In those cases, search for the general idea of the question.
Example:

> Which of the following was the psychological impact of the author's childhood upon the remainder of his life?

Key words are "childhood" or "psychology". While searching for those words, be alert for other words or phrases that have similar meaning, such as "emotional effect" or "mentally" which could be used in the passage, rather than the exact word "psychology".

Once you've quickly found the correct section of the passage to find the answer, focus upon the answer choices. Sometimes a choice will repeat word for word a portion of the passage near the answer. However, beware of such duplication – it may be a trap! More than likely, the correct choice will paraphrase or summarize the related portion of the passage, rather than being exactly the same wording.

For the answers that you think are correct, read them carefully and make sure that they answer the question. An answer can be factually correct, but it MUST answer the question asked. Additionally, two answers can both be seemingly correct, so be sure to read all of the answer choices, and make sure that you get the one that BEST answers the question.

Questions with no key word
Example:

> Which of the following would the author of this passage likely agree with?

In these cases, look for key words in the answer choices. Then skim the passage to find where the answer choice occurs. By skimming to find where to look, you can minimize the time required.

Sometimes it may be difficult to identify a good key word in the question to skim for in the passage. In those cases, look for a key word in one of the answer choices to skim for. Often the answer choices can all be found in the same paragraph, which can quickly narrow your search.

Paragraph Focus

Focus upon the first sentence of each paragraph, which is the most important. The main topic of the paragraph is usually there. Once you've read the first sentence in the paragraph, you have a general idea about what each paragraph will be about. As you read the questions, try to determine which paragraph will have the answer. Paragraphs have a concise topic. Whether the answer is there or not should be obvious. It will save time if you can jump straight to the paragraph, so try to remember what you learned from the first sentences.

Main idea
A reader has found the main idea when they understand the most important point the author is making. Readers must be able to read a short or long passage and distill the information into a single idea. A reader can review a multi-paragraph passage and find the main idea of each paragraph. Once the main idea of each paragraph is identified, the reader should be able to recognize a recurring or cohesive theme. If a test question asks a student to select the main idea of a passage from four possible answer choices, the student can do so by counting the number of paragraphs in which each answer choice is mentioned. The choice that is mentioned in most of the paragraphs is usually the correct answer.

For each answer choice, try to see how many paragraphs are related. It can help to count how many sentences are affected by each choice, but it is best to see how many paragraphs are affected by the choice. Typically the answer choices will include incorrect choices that are main ideas of individual paragraphs, but not the entire passage. That is why it is crucial to choose ideas that are supported by the most paragraphs possible.

> **Review Video: <u>Topics and Main Ideas</u>**
> *Visit **mometrix.com/academy**
> and enter Code*: **407801**

Writer's intent
Readers and writers perform their tasks with the same purposes: information or entertainment. A reader may read to be entertained or to gain information. Writers may write to inform or to entertain. Readers must be wary that sometimes writers can present an entertaining piece of writing as an informative piece. A writer may attempt to manipulate a reader by presenting their opinions as objective statements.

Readers must be able to distinguish a writer's purpose and tone in order to comprehend fully

the writer's intentions. A reader should ask themselves two questions:
  1) Who is the audience?
  2) Why is this being written?

A writer may be attempting to persuade the reader to act on something or think a certain way. A passage that contains words with either positive or negative connotations usually indicates that the writer is attempting to persuade a reader.

Supporting details
Supporting details are crucial to a story. These details allow the reader to "see" a character or scene in their mind. Supporting details may include descriptions of the weather, the color of a character's eyes or hair, or the sounds that a character hears. All of these details help readers understand the character as a person. Supporting details also add interest to a story. Readers must be able to distinguish between a main idea and supporting details. Supporting details are usually mentioned only once; they help create or develop the main idea.

> **Review Video: <u>Supporting Details</u>**
> *Visit **mometrix.com/academy**
> and enter Code*: **396297**

Context

On standardized tests (and in everyday life, for that matter) we are faced with words with which we are not familiar. In most cases, the definitions of these words can be derived from context clues. Context clues are the manner in which the word is used. When reading a passage, carefully look at the unfamiliar word or words. The author may provide a definition in parenthesis or a synonym for the unfamiliar word. Synonyms are useful, because they provide a common substitute for the unfamiliar word.

Authors may also provide an antonym, which is the opposite of the unfamiliar word. Another context clue may be a restatement of the idea that originally used an unfamiliar word. Sometimes, the author may even provide a detailed explanation of the unfamiliar word.

Eliminate Choices

Some choices can quickly be eliminated. "Anti-gout drugs are developed there." Is Gout even mentioned in the article? If not, quickly eliminate it.

When trying to answer a question such as "the passage indicates all of the following EXCEPT" quickly skim the paragraph searching for references to each choice. If the reference exists, scratch it off as a choice. Similar choices may be crossed off simultaneously if they are close enough.

Some choices will ask you to choose, "Which answer choice does NOT describe?" or "All of the following answer choices are identifiable characteristics, EXCEPT which one?" For these questions, look for answers that are similarly worded. Since only one answer can be correct, if there are two answers that appear to mean the same thing, they must BOTH be incorrect, and can be eliminated.

Example:

- A.) changing values and attitudes
- B.) a large population of mobile or uprooted people

These answer choices are similar; they both describe a fluid culture. Because of their similarity, they can be linked together. Since the answer can have only one choice, they can also be eliminated together.

Contextual Clues

Look for contextual clues. An answer can be *right* but not *correct*. The contextual clues will help you find the answer that is most right and is correct. Understand the context in which a phrase is stated.

When asked for the implied meaning of a statement made in the passage, immediately go find the statement and read the context it was made in. Also, look for an answer choice that has a similar phrase to the statement in question.

Example:

In the passage, what is implied by the phrase "Churches have become more or less part of the furniture"?

Find an answer choice that is similar or describes the phrase "part of the furniture" as that is the key phrase in the question. "Part of the furniture" is a saying that means something is fixed, immovable, or set in their ways. Those are all similar ways of saying "part of the furniture." As such, the correct answer choice will probably include a similar rewording of the expression.

Example:

Why was John described as "morally desperate"?

The answer will probably have some sort of definition of morals in it. "Morals" refers to a code of right and wrong behavior, so the correct answer choice will likely have words that mean something like that.

Fact/Opinion

A successful reader is able to interpret an author's intentions. Authors have many reasons for writing. It is the reader's job to understand the author's message. Every writer has their own values, opinions, and beliefs, and these are present in their writing. Readers must distinguish between the facts and opinions presented by a writer. A fact is a piece of information that can be proven, while an opinion is simply one person's view or belief. Opinions cannot be proven. A fact is objective, while an opinion is subjective. Concrete, measurable words often indicate a factual piece of information. Opinions are presented with judgmental or emotional terms. For example, the words best, worst, easiest, and ugliest usually describe subjective judgments, and therefore are more likely to appear in statements of opinion.

When asked about which statement is a fact or opinion, remember that answer choices that are facts will typically have no ambiguous words. For example, how long is a long time? What defines an ordinary person? These ambiguous words of "long" and "ordinary" should not be in a

factual statement. However, if all of the choices have ambiguous words, go to the context of the passage. Often a factual statement may be set out as a research finding.
Example:
"The scientist found that the eye reacts quickly to change in light."

Opinions may be set out in the context of words like thought, believed, understood, or wished.
Example:
"He thought the Yankees should win the World Series."

> ➤ **Review Video: Fact or Opinion**
> *Visit* **mometrix.com/academy**
> *and enter* **Code**: **870899**

Opposites

Answer choices that are direct opposites are usually correct. The paragraph will often contain established relationships (when this goes up, that goes down). The question may ask you to draw conclusions for this and will give two similar answer choices that are opposites.
Example:
A decrease in housing starts
An increase in housing starts

Make Predictions

As you read and understand the passage and then the question, try to guess what the answer will be. Remember that three of the four answer choices are wrong, and once you being reading them, your mind will immediately become cluttered with answer choices designed to throw you off. Your mind is typically the most focused immediately after you have read the passage and question and digested its contents. If you can, try to predict what the correct answer will be. You may be surprised at what you can predict.

Quickly scan the choices and see if your prediction is in the listed answer choices. If it is, then you can be quite confident that you have the right answer. It still won't hurt to check the other answer choices, but most of the time, you've got it!

Answer the Question

It may seem obvious to only pick answer choices that answer the question, but HESI A[2] exam can create some excellent answer choices that are wrong. Don't pick an answer just because it sounds right, or you believe it to be true. It MUST answer the question. Once you've made your selection, always go back and check it against the question and make sure that you didn't misread the question, and the answer choice does answer the question posed.

Benchmark

After you read the first answer choice, decide if you think it sounds correct or not. If it doesn't, move on to the next answer choice. If it does, make a mental note (or rest your pencil tip on the Scantron circle for choice A) about that choice. This doesn't mean that you've definitely selected it as your answer choice, it just means that it's the best you've seen thus far. Go ahead and read the next choice. If the next choice is worse than the one you've already selected, keep going to the next answer choice. If the next choice is better than the choice you've already selected, then make a mental note about that answer choice.

As you read through the list, you are mentally noting the choice you think is right. That is your new standard. Every other answer choice must be benchmarked against that standard. That choice is correct until proven otherwise by another answer choice beating it out. Once you've decided that no other answer choice seems as good, do one final check to ensure that it answers the question posed.

New Information

Correct answers will usually contain the information listed in the paragraph and question. Rarely will completely new information be inserted into a correct answer choice. Occasionally the new information may be related in a manner that HESI A[2] exam is asking for you to interpret, but seldom.

Example:
> The argument above is dependent upon which of the following assumptions: Charles's Law was used

If Charles's Law is not mentioned at all in the referenced paragraph and argument, then it is unlikely that this choice is correct. All of the information needed to answer the question is provided for you, and so you should not have to make guesses that are unsupported or choose answer choices that have unknown information that cannot be reasoned.

Valid Information

Don't discount any of the information provided in the passage, particularly shorter ones. Every piece of information may be necessary to determine the correct answer. None of the information in the paragraph is there to throw you off (while the answer choices will certainly have information to throw you off). If two seemingly unrelated topics are discussed, don't ignore either. You can be confident there is a relationship, or it wouldn't be included in the paragraph, and you are probably going to have to determine what that relationship is for the answer.

Logical inferences

Inferences are educated guesses that can be drawn from the facts and information available to a reader. Inferences are usually based upon a reader's own assumptions and beliefs. The ability to make inferences is often called reading between the lines. There are three basic types of inference: deductive reasoning, abductive reasoning, and inductive reasoning.

Deductive reasoning is the ability to find an effect when given a cause and a rule. Abductive reasoning is the ability to find a cause when given a rule and an effect. Inductive reasoning is the ability to find a rule when given the cause and effect. Each type of reasoning can be used to make logical inferences from a piece of writing.

Summarizing a passage

Summarizing a passage can seem like an overwhelming task, especially when the passage is long. Summarizing can help students to understand the main idea of a passage. It can also help a student to understand the author's tone and purpose. Summarizing a passage is a skill that must be practiced. Students can follow three basic rules when summarizing. First, list the main ideas from the beginning, middle, and end of the passage. Next, summarize the passage in sequence. In other words, do not skip around in the passage. Summarize from beginning to middle to end. The third rule is to make sure that the summary contains accurate information. Test questions may ask students to select the best summary of a passage. By using these three rules, students will be able to eliminate incorrect answers and select the best answer.

Time Management

In technical passages, do not get lost on the technical terms. Skip them and move on. You want a general understanding of what is going on, not a mastery of the passage.

When you encounter material in the selection that seems difficult to understand, it often may not be necessary and can be skipped. Only spend time trying to understand it if it is going to be relevant for a question. Understand difficult phrases only as a last resort.

Answer general questions before detail questions. A reader with a good understanding of the whole passage can often answer general questions without rereading a word. Get the easier questions out of the way before tackling the more time consuming ones.

Identify each question by type. Usually the wording of a question will tell you whether you can find the answer by referring directly to the passage or by using your reasoning powers. You alone know which question types you customarily handle with ease and which give you trouble and will require more time. Save the difficult questions for last.

Word Usage Questions

When asked how a word is used in the passage, don't use your existing knowledge of the word. The question is being asked precisely because there is some strange or unusual usage of the word in the passage. Go to the passage and use contextual clues to determine the answer. Don't simply use the popular definition you already know.

> ➤ **Review Video: Context**
> Visit *mometrix.com/academy*
> *and enter Code: 613660*

Switchback Words

Stay alert for "switchbacks." These are the words and phrases frequently used to alert you to shifts in thought. The most common switchback word is "but." Others include although, however, nevertheless, on the other hand, even though, while, in spite of, despite, regardless of.

Avoid "Fact Traps"

Once you know which paragraph the answer will be in, focus on that paragraph. However, don't get distracted by a choice that is factually true about the paragraph. Your search is for the answer that answers the question, which may be about a tiny aspect in the paragraph. Stay focused and don't fall for an answer that describes the larger picture of the paragraph. Always go back to the question and make sure you're choosing an answer that actually answers the question and is not just a true statement.

Vocabulary and General Knowledge

The Vocabulary and General Knowledge exam has 50 items, and contains basic vocabulary that is often used in health care fields. Time allotment: 50 minutes.

Increasing verbal ability

Nursing, like many professions, requires the ability to communicate effectively. Students should prepare for standardized testing and their nursing careers by utilizing some basic techniques for increasing vocabulary. Writing down new words is a good way to increase vocabulary. While reading, watching TV, or talking to others, make a note of any unfamiliar words you encounter. Look up the definition of those words and then attempt to use them in conversation. This will help the word become part of your general store of knowledge. Reading new and different material will also increase vocabulary. For example, if you normally read fashion magazines, try thumbing through a professional journal of archaeology or mathematics. This will introduce new words that you would not encounter in everyday life. Playing games like Scrabble and solving crossword puzzles can also help build verbal ability.

Etymology

Etymology is the study of words. It specifically focuses on the origins of words: how they have developed over time and between languages. Language is made up of words from different cultures and areas of the world. Some words we use today mean something completely different from what they meant hundreds of years ago. Words are constantly being redefined, changed, and created. New words appear as technology increases. Some words are formed by combining root words with prefixes and suffixes. Students who must improve verbal ability for standardized testing can do so by studying common prefixes and suffixes. By understanding the prefix pre, a student increases their chances of understanding words like predate. The prefix pre means "before", so it can be reasoned that predate means to date something in advance, such as predating a check.

Glossary of Important Terms

A

Abrasion-injury to the integrity of the skin resulting in skin loss

Abrupt- describes a sudden change that occurs without warning

Abscess-pus forming a pocket

Abstain- the deliberate effort to refrain from an action, such as drinking alcohol or eating junk food

Acapnia-low level of carbon dioxide in the blood

Accept- to willingly receive something; the process of granting approval

Access- the freedom to use something as one chooses; the permission or ability to enter or approach a specific entity or area

Accountable- responsible for actions or explanations

Acne-inflammation of the skin related to glands and hair

Adenoiditis-inflammation of the adenoids

Adhere- the process of binding one thing to another using glue, tape, or another agent; refers to the action of maintaining loyalty or support

Adverse- in a contrary fashion; can cause harm; may also refer to something that is in opposition to one's interests

Alopecia-bald condition

Amenorrhea-no menstrual discharge

Annual- the duration of a single year; an occurrence that takes place once each year

Anorchism-absence of testis

Anoxia-deficiency of oxygen

Anterior-frontal position

Anteroposterior-frontal to back positioning

Anuria-no urine production

Aphonia-no voice

Apnea-not breathing

Apply- to put something to use; having a relevant or valid connection to something else

Atelectasis-abnormal expansion of a lung

Audible- capable of being heard

Azoturia-elevated and excessive level of nitrogen substrates and urea in the urine

B

Balanitis-inflammation of the penis

Balanorrhea-elevated discharge of the penis

Bilateral- having two sides; may refer to something that affects both side of the human body

Biopsy-removal of tissue for evaluation purposes

Bronchogram-x-ray of the bronchi

Bronchography-the taking of the bronchi x-ray

C

Carbuncle-skin disease associated with boils

Carcinogen-cancer causing agent

Carcinoma-malignant tumor

Cast- the process by which something is given shape through the pouring of a liquid substance into a mold; may also refer to the throwing of an object

Caudal-related to the tail position

Cease- to bring about a gradual end; refers to something that dies out or becomes extinct

Cellulitis- inflammation of connective tissue, associated with infection and fever

Cephalic-related to the head position

Cervicectomy-removal of the cervix

Cicatrix-scar

Colpoplasty-repair of the vagina

Colposcope-device used to explore the vagina and cervix with visual examination

Compensatory- an equivalent; the action of making a payment that serves as a counterbalance for another action

Complications- a factor that presents a degree of difficulty; may also refer to a secondary disease or condition

Comply- to carry out the wishes of another person; to perform in the manner prescribed by law

Concave- a surface that is rounded inward like a bowl; surface that is arched or curved

Concise- straightforward and to the point; absent of all excessive detail

Consistency- the agreement of each of the parts that constitute a whole

Constrict- to make something narrow by squeezing or compressing

Contingent- something that may happen; may also refer to something that is dependent upon or conditioned by something else

Contour- the line that represents the shape of a curvy figure

Contract- an agreement between two parties that binds each to perform certain actions

Contraindication- the presence of a symptom or condition that will make a specific treatment unadvisable

Contusion-bruising of tissue with no loss in skin integrity

Cyanosis-bluish color of the skin related to poor blood supply

Cystogram-x-ray of the bladder

Cystoscope-device used for inspection of the bladder

Cystoscopy-examination of the bladder by vision

Cytogenic-related to the creation of cells

Cytoid-similar to a cell

Cytology-study of cellular biology

Cytoplasm-element inside the cell

D

Debridement-removal of necrotic tissue from a wound

Decubitus ulcer-wound related to a bedsore

Deficit- a lack in an amount or quality of something, such as money or rainfall

Depress- to press down; the lessening of activity or strength; an action in which something moves to a lower position

Depth- a quality of being complete and thorough

Dermatitis-inflammation of the dermis

Dermatoconiosis-aberrant condition of the epidermis created by dust

Dermatofibroma-skin tumor caused by fibrous cells

Dermatologist-doctor that focuses on skin condition/treatment

Dermatology-study of skin

Dermatome-surgical device for skin surgery

Dermatoplasty-surgery involving the skin

Deteriorating- to make inferior in quality; to diminish in function or condition

Device- something that is devised or thought up; may be a piece of equipment designed for a specific task

Diagnosis-determining the dysfunction/disease

Diameter- the length of a line that passes through the body of an object

Dilate- to enlarge, extend, or widen; to become wide like the pupil of the eye

Dilute- to make a substance thinner or less potent; diminish in flavor or intensity

Discrete- a separate entity; unique and separate from other things

Distal-away from a point of origin

Distended- something that has been enlarged by the force of internal pressure

Distinct- something that the eye or mind can easily separate from something else; something that is notable in its difference from other things

Dorsal-related to a rear position

Dyspareunia-painful sexual intercourse

Dysphonia-trouble with speaking

Dysplasia-aberrant development

Dyspnea-breathing complications

Dysuria-urination that is painful

E

Elevate- to lift or make something higher; to lift in rank or title

Endogenous- the growth from a deep tissue; refers to conditions that arise from factors that are internal to an organism

Endoscopy-inspection of a body cavity with visual examination

Enuresis-uncontrollable urination

Epidermal-related to the skin

Epididymitis-inflammation of the epididymis

Epithelial-related to epithelium tissue

Epithelioma-tumor made of skin cells

Erythema-redness in a appearance

Erythrocyte-red blood cell

Erythrocytosis- elevated red blood cell count

Erythroderma-redness of the skin

Etiology-study of disease relationships/origin

Eupnea-normal breathing

Exacerbate- to cause something to become more intense in nature; especially an increase in violence or severity

Excess- surpassing usual limitations; unnecessary indulgence

Exogenous- the growth from superficial or shallow tissue; refers to conditions caused by factors that are external to an organism

Expand- to open or unfold; refers to an increase in number, size, or scope; may refer to the expression of an idea in greater depth

Exposure- being subject to a condition or influence; making a secret fact known publicly

External- being outside the human body; existing outside the confines of a specific space or institution

F

Fatal- something that may cause death; relating to fate or proceeding in a manner that follows a fixed sequence of events

Fatigue- the state of tiredness brought on by labor, exertion, or stress; the tendency of a specified material to break under stress

Fibroma-tumor made of fibrous cells

Fibrosarcoma-malignant tumor made of fibrous cells

Fissure-crack in the skin's integrity

Flaccid- the state of not being firm; lacking vigor, force, or youthful firmness

Flush- to chase from a place of concealment; forcing one substance out of a space by introducing another substance

G

Gaping- something that is wide open and exposed

Gender- the behavioral, cultural, or psychological traits that are associated with a specific sex

H

Hepatosalpinx-fallopian tube with blood present

Hidradenitis-inflammation of sweat glands

Histology-study of tissues in nature

HIV-retrovirus that causes AIDS

Hydration- the taking up of elements with the aid of water; the constant supply of water or fluids

Hydrosalpinx-water in the fallopian tube

Hygiene- the science of health-inducing practices; the condition or practice of activities that can maintain physical health

Hymenectomy-removal of the hypmen

Hyperplasia-elevated numbers of cells

Hypocapnia-decreased level of carbon dioxide in the bloodstream

Hypodermic-related to underneath the skin

Hypoplasia-decreased numbers of cells required for normal organ development

Hypoxemia-limited oxygen in the bloodstream

Hysteropexy-fixation of the uterus

I

Iatrology-study of medicine

Impaired- a condition in which one cannot perform or function properly; often refers to a person who is under the influence of drugs or alcohol

Impending- hanging overhead threateningly; bound to occur in the near future

Incidence- the arrival of something at a surface; something that occurs or affects something else

Induration-firm point or points, possibly in the periwound area

Inferior-below a point of origin

Inflamed- to incite an intensely emotional state; also refers to something that has been set on fire

Ingest- to take into one's mouth for digestion

Initiate- to cause something to begin or to set events in motion; as initiation, can also refer to the process through which a person is allowed entry into a club or organization

Insidious- something or someone who is enticing but dangerous; slow-developing dangerousness

Intact- something that remains whole or untouched by destructive forces; having no relevant part removed or altered

Internal- things inside of the body or the mind; something that exists within the limits and confines of something else

Invasive- tending to spread or infringe upon something; may also refer to something that will enter the human body

K

Karyocyte- cellular unit with a nucleus

Keloid-scar tissue that has exhibited excessive growth

Keratogenic-creation of horny like tissue appearance

L

Labile- unstable; constantly undergoing a chemical or physical change or breakdown

Laceration-wound with irregular borders, knife like in appearance

Latent- not presently active but with the potential to become active

Lateral-opposite of medial, related to point of origin

Leiodermia- smooth skin

Leiomyoma-tumor made of smooth muscle cells

Leiomyosarcoma-malignant tumor made of smooth muscle cells
Lethargic- sluggish, indifferent, or apathetic
Leukocyte-white blood cell
Leukocytosis-elevated white blood cell count
Lipoid-fat like substance
Lipoma-tumor composed of fat
Liposarcoma-malignant tumor made of fat cells
Lithotripsy-crushing of a stone
Lumbar-lower back region

M
Mammogram-x-ray of the breast
Mammoplasty-repair of the breasts
Mammotome-device used to cut breast tissue
Manifestation- the act of becoming outwardly visible; can refer to the occult phenomenon of a supernatural materialization
Mastitis-inflammation of breast tissue
Mastectomy-removal of a breast
Mastoptosis-drooping breast
Menarche-start of menstruation
Menometrorrhagia-flow of blood during menstruation, and between cycles
Melanocarcinoma-malignant black tumor
Melanoma-tumor of the epithelial tissue
Metastasis-progression of a disease between organs, uncontrollable
Metrorrhea-uterus discharge that is excessive
Micturate-voiding or urination
Myometritis-inflammation of the uterine tissue
Myopathy-muscular disease

N
Necrosis-cellular death, often resulting in black, dead tissue
Neopathy- new-sprung disease
Nephrectomy-removal of a kidney
Nephrogram-x-ray of the kidney
Nephrolysis-kidney separation
Nephropexy-fixation of the kidney
Nephroma- kidney tumor
Nephromegaly-kidney enlargement
Nephroptosis- sagging kidney
Nephrostomy-creating an opening to the kidney
Neuroma-tumor involving nerves
Nocturia-urination at night
Nutrient- something that provides nourishment

O
Occluded- closed or blocked off
Oligomenorrhea-limited menstrual discharge
Ominous- exhibiting an omen; refers to something evil or disastrous that appears likely to occur
Oncology-study of tumor like tissue
Ongoing- in the process of occurring; continuously advancing or moving ahead
Onychectomy- removal of a nail
Onychomycosis-fungal condition in the nail
Onychophagia-eating your nails
Onychopryptosis-ingrown nail
Oophorectomy-removal of an ovary
Oophoritis-inflammation of the ovary
Oral- spoken by the mouth; of or relating to the mouth
Orchidectomy-removal of both or one testis
Orchidotomy-incision made into the testis
Orchiepididymitis-inflammation of the epididymis and testis
Orchioplasty-repair of the testis
Orchitis-inflammation of the testicle
Overt- something that is openly displayed or obvious
Oximeter-a device used to measure oxygen saturation of the blood

P
Pachyderma-increased thickness of the skin
Parameter- a limit or boundary; in math, it is an arbitrary value that is used to describe a statistical population
Paroxysmal- characterized by a sudden fit or attack of symptoms; may be a sudden emotion or uncontrollable action
Paroxysm-sudden attack
Patent- a proprietary statement; conveys ownership of an idea or invention; being granted a free and easily accessible passage
Pathogenic-disease causing
Pathologist-individual who studies pathology
Pediculosis-condition of lice
Percutaneous- penetrating the skin
Pleuritis-inflammation of the pleura
Pneumatocele-hernia associated with the lung
Pneumoconiosis-dust in the lung's condition
Pneumonia-disease of the lung related to infection
Pneumothorax-air in the chest resulting in the collapse of a lung

Posterior-related to the rear/back position

Potent- able to copulate as a male; refers to something that is chemically or medically effective

Potential- having the possibility of becoming a reality

Precaution- the act of taking care in advance; refers to measures taken in advance in order to prevent harm

Precipitous- very steep or difficult to climb or overcome

Predispose- to dispose in advance of or to make susceptible to

Preexisting- the state of existing before or previous to something else

Primary- first in order; a rank of importance

Priority- the state of being before; coming first in order of date or position; a preferential rating

Prognosis- the possibility of recovery after the diagnosis of an illness or disease

Prognosis-opinion of an individual about outcomes

Pruritus-uncontrollable itching

Pyelolithotomy-incision to remove a stone from the renal pelvis

Pyeloplasty-repair of the renal pelvis

Pyosalpinx-pus in the fallopian tube

Pyuria-pus in the urine

R

Rationale- an explanation regarding the principles, opinions, beliefs, or practices held by a specific party

Recur- something that is revisited for consideration; a thought or idea that enters one's mind for a second time

Restrict- to confine something or someone within specific limitations or boundaries

Retain- to keep in one's possession; to maintain an item or person in security

Rhabdomyosarcoma-tumor made of striated muscle cells

Rhinitis-inflammation of the nose

Rhinorrhagia-bleeding from the nose

Rhinorrhea-nose discharge

Rhytidectomy- removal of wrinkles in the skin

Rhytidoplasty- repair of wrinkles in the skin

S

Salpingocele-fallopian tube hernia

Sarcoma-tumor made up of connective tissue

Scleroderma-hardening of connective tissue, related to disease of various organs

Seborrhea-elevated production of sebum

Site- the physical location of a structure; the physical space reserved for a building; the place or scene of an occurrence

Somatic-related to the body

Somatopathy-disease related to the body

Somatoplasm-element of the body

Spirometer-device used to measure breathing capacity

Spirometry-taking a measurement of breathing capacity

Status- the position or rank held in relation to others; a person or object's condition with respect to circumstances

Strict- inflexible; maintained in such a manner that cannot be changed or altered

Subcutaneous-underneath the skin

Superior-elevated above a point of origin

Supplement- an item that completes something else

Suppress- to restrain by authority or force; to omit something from memory; to keep from public knowledge

Symmetric- exhibiting symmetry; capable of being divided by a longitudinal plane into equal sections

Symptom- the evidence of a disease or illness; the presence of a symptom is indicative of something else

Syphilis- a type of sexually transmitted disease

Systemic-throughout

T

Thoracalgia-pain located in the chest

Tracheitis-inflammation of the trachea

Tracheostenois- reduced trachea size

Trichomyosis-fungal condition in hair

U

Ungual-related to the nail

Unilateral- on one side of the body

Untoward- difficult to manage; marked by trouble or unpleasantness

Uremia-blood in the urine

Ureterectomy-removal of a ureter

Ureteritis-inflammation of the ureter

Ureterocele-ureter protrussion

Ureterolithiasis-stones in the ureter

Ureterostenosis-decreased diameter of the ureter
Urethrocystitis-inflammation of the bladder
Urinate- to expel urine
Urology-study of the urinary system

V

Vaginitis-inflammation of the vagina
Variocele-enlarged veins of the spermatic cord
Vasectomy-removal of a duct
Ventral-related to an anterior position
Verbal- relating to or consisting of words; involving words rather than meaning or substance
Visceral-related to the internal organ systems
Vital- necessary or essential to the existence of life
Void- not occupied or empty; of no legal force or effect
Volume- printed pages bound in a book form; space occupied by a three-dimensional form; degree of loudness
Vulvovaginitis-inflammation of the vagina and vulva

X

Xanthochromic-related to yellow coloring
Xanthoderma-jaundice like skin
Xanthosis-condition of yellow coloring present that is aberrant
Xeroderma- skin that is excessively dry

Grammar

Language

Prefixes

Prefixes are a group of letters that are placed in front of a root word. When combined with a root word, a prefix alters the meaning of the original word. For example, consider the prefix sub-. Sub- means under, below, or less than. Knowing this, one can combine the prefix sub- with a variety of root words and understand what each means. The word terrain refers to a piece of land or ground. By adding the word sub- to terrain one creates the word sub terrain. Based on the definition of each part of this word, one can assume that sub terrain refers to something that is below or underground.

> **Review Video: Prefixes**
> *Visit **mometrix.com/academy***
> *and enter **Code: 361382***

<u>Examples of some prefixes:</u>
The prefix a- means not or without. Words that use this prefix include amoral, atypical, and atheist.
The prefix ab- means away from. Words that use this prefix include abstain, abnormal, and absent.
The prefix ad- means toward or to. Words that use this prefix include addition, adhesive, and admonish.
The prefix ante- means before. Words that use this prefix include antemortem, antecedent, and antebellum.
The prefix anti- means against. Words that use this prefix include antidote, antibody, and antifreeze.
The prefix be- means by or near. Words that use this prefix include beside, begrudge, and belie.
The prefix bene- means good or well. Words that use this prefix include benefit, benevolent, and benediction.
The prefix bi- means two. Words that use this prefix include bilateral, bilingual, and bipartisan.
The prefix circum- means around or about. Words that use this prefix include circumnavigate, circumstantial, and circumference.
The prefix co- means with or together. Words that use this prefix include cosign, cooperate, and coworker.
The prefix com- means together. Words that use this prefix include combine, component, and compatible.
The prefix contra- means against. Words that use this prefix include contraband, contradict, and contrary.
The prefix counter- means opposite. Words that use this prefix include counterintelligence, counterintuitive, and counterproductive.
The prefix de- means from, down, or away. Words that use this prefix include degrade, despite, and detach.

The prefix equi- means equal. Words that use this prefix include equidistant, equivalent, and equinox.

The prefix ex- means out of or former. Words that use this prefix include exponent, extent, and examine.

The prefix extra- means beyond. Words that use this prefix include extraterrestrial, extraordinary, and extrasensory.

The prefix infra- means below or beneath. Words that use this prefix include infrastructure, infrared, and infrasonic.

The prefix inter- means between. Words that use this prefix include intercept, interoffice, and intercede.

The prefix intra- means within. Words that use this prefix include intravenous, intracranial, and intraorbital.

The prefix macro- means large. Words that use this prefix include macrobiotic, macrophage, and macroscopic.

The prefix mal- means bad. Words that use this prefix include malady, maladjusted, and malfunction.

The prefix mega- means large. Words that use this prefix include megaphone, megabyte, and megalopolis.

The prefix micro- means small. Words that use this prefix include microscope, micrometer, and microprocessor.

The prefix mid- means middle. Words that use this prefix include midday, midline, and midsummer.

The prefix mini- means small. Words that use this prefix include minivan, miniscule, and minimum.

The prefix mis- means wrong. Words that use this prefix include misfit, mismatch, and mistake.

The prefix multi- means many. Words that use this prefix include multicolor, multiply, and multinational.

The prefix non- means not. Words that use this prefix include nondescript, nonchalant, and nonfiction.

The prefix ob- means against. Words that use this prefix include object, obscure and obstinate.

The prefix over- means excessive. Words that use this prefix include overindulgent, overage, and oversensitive.

The prefix peri- means around. Words that use this prefix include perinatal, perimeter, and periscope.

The prefix poly- means many. Words that use this prefix include polynomial, polydactyl, and polygamy.

The prefix post- means after or later. Words that use this prefix include postmortem, posterior, and postlude.

The prefix pre- means before. Words that use this prefix include premonition, predecessor, and preeminent.

The prefix pro- means supporting. Words that use this prefix include probiotic, proliferate, and procreate.

The prefix pseudo- means false. Words that use this prefix include pseudonym, pseudonarcotic, and pseudomorph.

The prefix re- means again. Words that use this prefix include repeat, reverberate, and redirect.

The prefix retro- means backward. Words that use this prefix include retrofit, retrospect, and retroactive.

The prefix semi- means half. Words that use this prefix include semifinal, semiannual, and semicircle.

The prefix socio- means social or society. Words that use this prefix include sociopath, socioeconomic, and sociocultural.

The prefix sub- means under. Words that use this prefix include subject, subside, and submarine.

The prefix super- means above. Words that use this prefix include supernatural, supersede, and superficial.

The prefix supra- means above. Words that use this prefix include supraorbital, suprarenal, and supraliminal.

The prefix trans- means across. Words that use this prefix include transcontinental, transaction, and transvestite.

The prefix ultra- means beyond. Words that use this prefix include ultraviolet, ultrarapid, and ultrasafe.

The prefix un- means not. Words that use this prefix include undecided, unjust, and unforgettable.

The prefix under- means beneath. Words that use this prefix include underused, underage, and underlie.

The prefix tele- means from a distance or from afar. Words that use this prefix include telephone, telepathy, and teleport.

The prefix with- means against or back. Words that use this prefix include withhold, withstand, and withdraw.

The prefix neo- means new. Words that use this prefix include neoclassic, Neolithic, and neoplasm.

The prefix hyper- means over or above. Words that use this prefix include hypersensitive, hyperbole, and hypertext.

The prefix hypo- means below or less than. Words that use this prefix include hypoglycemia, hypothermia, and hypodermic.

The prefix in- means not. Words that use this prefix include insane, innate, and inorganic.

The prefix meso- means middle. Words that use this prefix include Mesolithic, mesosphere, and mesoderm.

The prefix syn- means together. Words that use this prefix include synergy, synthesis, and synchronize.

The prefix para- means beside. Words that use this prefix include paranormal, parametric, and paraprofessional.

The prefix phot- means light. Words that use this prefix include photograph, photosynthesize, and photon.

The prefix sanct- means holy. Words that use this prefix include sanction, sanctuary, and sanctimonious.

The prefix therm- means heat. Words that use this prefix include thermal, thermodynamic, and thermometer.

The prefix acro- means high, top, or tip. Words that use this prefix include acrophobia, acronym, and acrobat.

The prefix alt- means high. Words that use this prefix include altitude, altar, and altimeter.

The prefix audi- means to hear. Words that use this prefix include audible, audience, and audition.

The prefix auto- means self. Words that use this prefix include autobiography, autoimmune, and automotive.

The prefix vita- means life. Words that use this prefix include vitamins, vital, and vitalism.

The prefix chron- means time. Words that use this prefix include chronology, chronic, and chronicle.

The prefix ecto- means outside or external. Words that use this prefix include ectoplasm, ectosphere, and ectopic.

The prefix demo- means people. Words that use this prefix include demographic, demonstrate, and democracy.

The prefix dia- means through, across, or between. Words that use this prefix include diameter, diagonal, and diaphragm.

The prefix dis- means away, not, or negative. Words that use this prefix include dissuade, disengage, and disdain.

The prefix dyn- means power. Words that use this prefix include dynamic, dynasty, and dynamite.

The prefix endo- means inside. Words that use this prefix include endoscopic, endothermal, and endogenous.

The prefix omni- means all. Words that use this prefix include omnipotent, omniscient, and omnivorous.

The prefix homo- means same. Words that use this prefix include homogenous, homosexual, and homonym.

The prefix hetero- means other. Words that use this prefix include heterosexual, heterogony, and heterochromatic.

Suffixes

Suffixes are a group of letters placed behind a root word. Suffixes can perform one of two possible functions: they can be used to create a new word or they can shift the tense of a word without changing its original meaning. For example, the suffix -ability can be added to the end of the word account to form the new word accountability. Account means a written narrative or description of events, while accountability means the state of being liable. The suffix -ed can be added to account to form the word accounted, which simply shifts the word from present tense to past tense.

➤ **Review Video: Suffixes**
Visit ***mometrix.com/academy***
and enter ***Code: 212541***

Adding suffixes

Sometimes adding a suffix can change the spelling of a word. If the suffix begins with a vowel, the final consonant of the root word must be doubled. This rule applies only if the root word has one syllable or if the accent is on the last syllable. For example, when adding the suffix -ery to the root word rob, the final word becomes robbery. The letter b is doubled because rob is only one syllable. However, when adding the suffix -able to the root word profit, the final word becomes profitable. The letter t is not doubled because the root word profit has two syllables. Spelling is not changed when the suffixes -less, -ness, -ly, or -en are used. The only exception to this rule is when the root word ends in y and the suffix -ness or -ly will be added. In this case, the y changes to an i. For example, happy becomes happily.

Certain suffixes require that the root word be modified. If the suffix begins with a vowel, such as -ing, and the root word ends in the letter e, the letter e must be dropped before adding the suffix. For example, the word write will become writing. If the suffix begins with a consonant instead of a vowel, the letter e at the end of the root word does not need to be dropped. For example, hope would become hopeless. The only exceptions to this specific rule are the words judgment, acknowledgment, and argument. If a root word ends in the letter y and is preceded by a consonant, change the y to an i before adding the suffix. This is the case for all suffixes, except those that begin with the letter i. For example, plenty becomes plentiful.

Examples of suffixes

Suffix	Meaning	Sample words
-ability	having an inclination for	predictability, culpability, deniability
-able	worthy of an act	conceivable, valuable, laughable
-ac	pertaining to	cardiac, insomniac, maniac
-acy	having the quality of	efficacy, accuracy, democracy
-age	a collection or condition	bondage, footage, percentage
Suffix	Meaning	Sample words
-al	related to or process of	congenital, spatial, subliminal
-ance	the condition of	continuance, dominance, compliance
-ate	having	satiate, radiate, alienate
-ation	the process of or action	duplication, contamination, starvation
-cy	the condition or state of	pregnancy, bankruptcy, supremacy
-ed	the past tense of a verb	walked, cried, dated
-en	to cause to be	blacken, weaken, tighten
-ence	the state or condition of	independence, emergence, existence
-er	one who performs	dancer, entertainer, server
-ery	the state or place of	surgery, nunnery, bribery
-ese	relating to or having the characteristics of	legalese, Japanese, Balinese
-ial	pertaining to	colonial, tutorial, spatial
-ian	relating or belonging to	median, physician, statistician
-ing	conveys an action	calling, telling, shopping
-ist	one who performs an action	pianist, typist, sadist
-ious	full of or having	precocious, noxious, vicious
-ish	characteristic of	prudish, Amish, foolish

- 21 -

Suffix	Meaning	Examples
-ism	action or practice of	alcoholism, fascism, terrorism
-ity	the action or process of	abnormality, partiality, oddity
-ive	performing an action	impassive, decisive, demonstrative
-ize	to cause to be	immobilize, standardize, prioritize
-less	without	powerless, joyless, fearless
-logy	study of	theology, psychology, archaeology
-ment	action or process of	merriment, banishment, replacement
-meter	measurement of	thermometer, perimeter, centimeter
-ness	quality or condition	fullness, happiness, sadness
-oid	resembling	humanoid, asteroid, spheroid
-or	state of	behavior, demeanor, fervor
-ory	characterized by	auditory, statutory, mandatory
-ose	full of or possessing	varicose, comatose, sucrose
-osis	conveys a condition	mitosis, osmosis, neurosis
-s/-es	indicates that a word is plural	tomatoes, wagons, boys
-ship	the state or quality of	hardship, ownership, apprenticeship
-some	full of	lonesome, worrisome, tiresome
-tion	an action or condition	contrition, abolition, superstition
-ty	quality or condition of	vanity, sanctity, loyalty
-cide	to kill	infanticide, fratricide, genocide
-ectomy	to cut away	mastectomy, vasectomy, appendectomy
-ite	one connected with	graphite, trilobite, hematite
-ia	an act or state	insomnia, mania, hypoglycemia
-phobia	illogical fear of	aquaphobia, arachnophobia, claustrophobia

Root words:

Root	Meaning	Examples
ac	to do	action, active, activity
ag	to do	agenda, agree, agitate
agri	farm	agriculture, agribusiness
anthropo	man	anthropology, anthropomorphic
aqua	water	aquatic, aquaphilia
aud	hearing	audio, auditory
auto	self	autopilot, autopsy
biblio	book	bibliography, biblioclast
bio	life	biology, biometrics
capit	head	capital, capitulate
cede	go	recede, intercede
celer	speed	accelerate, decelerate
chron	time	chronology, chronic
cide	kill	infanticide, pesticide
clued	close	include, preclude, conclude
cog	knowledge	cognizant, precognition
ded	give	dedicate
dent	tooth	dental, dentist

duc	lead	induct, induce	psych	mind	psychology, psychic
fac	make or do	manufacture, facilitate	reg	rule	regulate, regal
fer	carry	ferry, transfer	rupt	break	interrupt, rupture
fract	break	fracture, fraction	Sect	cut	section, sector
frater	brother	fraternity, fraternal	Sert	bind	insert
gen	produce	generate, antigen	scend	climb	descend, ascend
geo	earth	geography, geology	scribe	write	prescribe, describe
graph	picture or writing	epigraph, pictograph	spect	look at	spectator, spectacle
hemo	blood	hemoglobin, hemophilia	Spir	breath	respiration, respiratory
homo	man	homogenous, homicide	strict	tighten	constrict, restrict
hydr	water	hydraulic, hydration	Tain	hold	detain, abstain
ject	throw	trajectory, inject	Term	end	terminal, terminate
jud	right	judge, judicial	tract	draw	retract, traction
junct	join	junction, conjunctivitis	typ	print	typical, typewriter
juris	justice or law	jurisdiction	Ven	come	convene, venue
lect	read	lecture, elect	Vict	conquer	victory, evict
logue	speech	dialogue, monologue	Vis	see	vision, visit
loq	speak	soliloquy	Volt	turn	revolt
lude	play	interlude, delude	alter	other	alternate, alternative
manu	hand	manuscript, manual	Ami	love	amiable
mand	order	commander, reprimand	amphi	all sides	amphibian, amphitheater
mater	mother	maternal, matriarch	Ann	year	annual, anniversary
mort	death	mortuary, mortician	arch	leader	archangel, monarch
mute	change	mutation, commute	Bell	war	belligerent, bellow
naut	sailor or ship	nautical, astronaut	brev	short	abbreviate, brevity
nounce	declare	announce, pronounce	Cap	take or seize	capture, captive
ped	foot	pedicure, pedal	carn	meat	carnivore, carnage
philo	love	philosophy, hydrophilia	Ced	yield or go	recede, precede
port	carry	portal, porter	chrom	color	chromatic, monochrome
			corp	body	corporal, corpse
			Crat	ruler	autocrat, aristocrat
			Cred	believe	incredible, credulous

cruc	cross	crucial, crucify
crypt	hidden	cryptic, cryptogram
Culp	guilt	culprit, culpable
Dei	god	deity, deify
derm	skin	epidermal, dermatologist
Dic	speak	dictionary, indict
Dox	belief or opinion	paradox, orthodox
gress	step	progress, ingress
Gyn	woman	gynecology, androgyny
Holo	whole, entire	holograph, holistic
Iso	equal, identical	isometric, isolate
Liter	letter	literate, literary
Loc	place	local, location
magn	large	magnum, magnify
meta	behind, between	metatarsal, metaphysics
Mit	send	permit, emit
Mon	warn	admonish, premonition
neuro	nerve	neuron, neurology
Nov	new	novel, renovate
onym	word, name	synonym, acronym
Pac	peace	pacify, pact
pater	father	paternal, patriarch
Path	suffering	sympathy, pathology
Puls	push	impulse, pulsate
pend	hang, weigh	suspend, pendant
phon	sound, voice	phonetics, telephone
Plan	flat	planar, plantation
pugna	fight	pugilist, repugnant
quer	ask	query, inquisition
simil	same	similar, simile
Sol	Sun	solar, solarium
Son	sound	sonar, unison
soph	knowledge	sophisticate, philosophy
spond	promise	respond
Stat	position	static, station
temp	time	temporal, temperature
Terr	Earth	terrain, terrestrial
trophy	nutrition or food	atrophy, dystrophy
ver	truth	verify, veritable
Vac	empty	vacuum, vacate

Antonyms

Some words have similar meanings, and some words have opposite meanings. An antonym is a pair of words that mean the opposite of each other. Examples are hot and cold, high and low, in and out, over and under, up and down, stop and start, good and bad, long and short, fast and slow, live and die, fat and skinny, happy and sad, content and displeased, shallow and deep, loose and tight, hard and soft, break and repair, inflate and deflate, ugly and pretty, and forget and remember. Not all words have antonyms. Some words, such as nouns, are non-opposable. For example, the word giraffe has no antonym. Some words can be turned into their own antonym by adding the prefix un-. For example, real and unreal, done and undone, settle and unsettle, and tie and untie.

> **Review Video:**
> **Synonyms and Antonyms**
> Visit *mometrix.com/academy*
> and enter **Code: 105612**

Synonyms

Synonyms are words that share the same or similar meanings. Synonyms can be substitutes for one another while preserving the meaning of a phrase. One word can have several synonyms. Synonyms are a useful tool because they allow one to incorporate variation into their writing or speaking. Instead of using the same word repeatedly, synonyms can be incorporated. Synonyms for the word many include several, a lot, myriad, and numerous. Synonyms for practical include handy, useful, and functional. Synonyms for walk include ambulate, foot, pace, and tread. Synonyms for happy include chipper, lighthearted, sunny, bright, and cheery. Synonyms for distress include concern, trouble, and worry.

➢ **Review Video:**
Synonmys and Antonyms Continued
Visit mometrix.com/academy
and enter Code: **440473**

Analogies

Analogies are based on logical assumptions. They test a student's ability to use reasoning and critical thinking when solving a problem. Analogies require students to think about and analyze a problem in order to find the solution. Verbal analogies will require the student to select the missing term and the analogies will be presented in one of five formats. Every analogy contains four terms in a specific order. Any one of the terms can be missing. Or, in another format, the second pair of terms may be omitted. A completed question may look like this: Laugh : Cry :: Happy : Sad. When presented on the test, one of the terms may be omitted-- Laugh : Cry :: Happy : _____. A pair of word omissions would look like this: Laugh : Cry :: _____. There will be four possible answers.

Example:
> From the following analogies, select the pair that has opposite meaning and explain:
> A) Heavy-Solid
> B) Touch-Feel
> C) Artificial-Real
> D) Similar-Alike

The pair that has opposite meaning is choice C. The words are antonyms: they have opposite meanings. Artificial means fake or having unrealistic qualities, while real means exactly the opposite. The other pairs are all synonyms. Heavy and solid both convey the sense that an object that has significant weight. The pair touch and feel can be used to describe the act of using one's hands to explore an object. The pair similar

and alike are synonyms that can be used to describe items that share the same qualities.

On a standardized test, analogies are grouped according to subject matter. There are six possible subject areas: social science, natural science, mathematics, humanities, English grammar and usage, and commonplace knowledge. Social science questions will use terms that relate to areas such as government, history, geography, and psychology. Natural science questions will use terms relating to areas such as astronomy, biology, and physics. Mathematics analogies will use numbers, patterns, and sequences. Humanities content will include terms relating to areas such as performing arts, literature, and religion. English grammar and usage analogies will feature terms that include parts of speech, punctuation, and style. Commonplace knowledge will feature analogies from everyday life.

Several basic relationship patterns appear within analogy questions. Once a test taker can recognize these patterns, they increase their chances of answering the question correctly. One pattern is the part-to-whole analogy, in which one term is a component of the other term. For example, finger is to hand as toe is to foot. The pattern may also appear in the other direction as a whole-to-part analogy: hand is to finger as foot is to toe. Another common pattern is the cause-and-effect analogy. For example, fire is to burn as ice is to freeze. Fire causes things to burn, while ice causes things to freeze. Another pattern is the defining characteristic analogy, in which one term represents a quality or characteristic of the other term. For example, swimming is to fish as flying is to bird.

Another common relationship a student may see in an analogy is the synonym relationship. One term will have the same or almost the same definition as the other. For example, rot is to decay as fix is to repair. Conversely, there is the antonym pattern, in which the terms have opposite meanings. For example, break is to repair as high is to low. Another pattern found within analogies is the sequence pattern. This pattern presents terms in a sequential order. For example, spring is to summer as fall is to winter.

In these pairs, the first terms precede the second terms in seasonal order. Another pattern is the degree-of-intensity pattern. Each term will represent a degree of intensity of the same concept. For example, interest is to obsession as like is to love. The terms interest and like are milder forms of the terms obsession and love.

In member and class analogies, one term represents a component of the class described by the other term. For example, nonfiction is to literature as minivan is to automobile. Definition analogies feature terms that describe one another. For example, blender is to mix as stove is to cook. You may define a blender as a tool to mix things, while a stove is a tool to cook things. A manner analogy features one verb that explains how another verb is performed. For example, blubber is to cry as saunter is to walk. The lack-of analogy features one term that describes the absence of the other term. For example, hotheaded is to patience as dry is to water. The term hotheaded means a lack of patience, while the term dry means something lacks water or moisture.

In a functional analogy, one term describes the purpose or function of the other. For example, stethoscope is to heartbeat as telescope is to constellation. In action-and-significance analogies, one term describes an action while the other indicates the significance of that action. For example, applaud is to approval as yawn is to tiredness. Another pattern in analogies is the pertinence relationship. In this type of analogy one term represents, or pertains to, a specific type of the class described by the other term. For example, Times New Roman is to font as watercolor is to paint.

Some analogies have a symbol and representation relationship, in which one term is the symbol that represents the other term. For example, red is to stop as green is to go. Or cross is to holy as clover is to lucky. Another relationship is that of agent and action. One term is the agent that carries out the action. For example, eye is to seeing as ear is to hearing. In a component-and-product analogy, one term is a component or part of the other. For example, wax is to candle as wood is to tree.

Parts of Speech

Sentences

Phrases are groups of words that function as a single unit within a sentence. They do not contain a distinct subject or predicate. They can act as nouns, adjective, or adverbs.
A *sentence* is a complete thought that contains an identifiable subject and predicate.
A *subject* tells whom or what a sentence concerns.
A *predicate* includes a verb and tells what the subject does or what is done to the subject.
A *predicate adjective* follows a linking verb and reveals more information about the subject.
A *predicate nominative* is a noun or pronoun that follows a linking verb and further explains the subject.

Subject-verb agreement
Subjects and verbs must agree in number. This is a common mistake made by students, especially those rushing to complete a test. Avoid this mistake by first identifying the subject and the verb in a sentence. Make sure that the subject and verb agree in number, even if they are separated. Singular subjects require singular verbs, while plural subjects require plural verbs. Sometimes, a subject will be a collective noun representing a group. If the group acts as a single being, use a singular verb. If the group acts separately, use a plural verb. When there are two subjects separated by the word and, use a plural verb. When multiple subjects are separated by or, either/or, or neither/nor, use a singular verb.

> ➤ **Review Video:**
> **Subject-Verb Agreement**
> *Visit* **mometrix.com/academy**
> *and enter* **Code: 479190**

Commas in compound sentences
Compound sentences are sentences that contain two or more independent clauses. Independent clauses are simple sentences—they contain a subject and a predicate, and express a complete thought. Two independent clauses can be joined with a coordinating conjunction, such as but,

and, or, or nor. When this occurs, a comma must be placed before the coordinating conjunction. Make sure that the clauses are both independent before placing a comma in the sentence.

Run-on sentences

A run-on sentence exists when two or more sentences are strung together to form one long sentence. Run-on sentences can be corrected easily by adding the appropriate punctuation. A run-on can be separated into multiple sentences, or words can be added or altered to form a coherent sentence. A comma splice is a common type of error that leads to run-on sentences. A comma splice occurs when two independent clauses are joined by a comma. Two independent clauses should be separated by a dash, colon, or semicolon. Coordinating conjunctions can also be used to eliminate run-ons.

> ➢ **Review Video:**
> **Fragments and Run-on Sentences**
> *Visit **mometrix.com/academy***
> *and enter **Code: 541989***

Pronoun case

Pronoun case is the form of the noun or pronoun that indicates its relation to the other words in a sentence. The three pronoun cases are nominative, possessive, and objective. A pronoun's case is determined by how it is used in a sentence. Pronouns may be used as a subject, as an object of a preposition, or as a replacement for a possessive noun. When the pronoun is the subject of a sentence, use the nominative form, such as I, he, or she. When the pronoun is the object of a preposition, use the objective form, such as them. When the pronoun replaces a possessive noun, use the possessive form, such as his or hers.

Commas in a series

Commas should be placed between all the elements in a series. A series consists of at least three items. The items may be single words, phrases, or clauses. Consider this example: I bought milk, juice, apples, and cereal. There are four items in the series. Each item is followed by a comma, including the item before the conjunction. This helps to avoid confusion. Some

authorities say that it is optional to insert a comma before a conjunction. In most cases, the addition of a comma between a series item and the conjunction can help to avoid confusion.

Nouns

A noun is a word that refers to a person, place, or thing. A noun may also refer to an idea. The four types of nouns include proper nouns, common nouns, abstract nouns, and collective nouns. Proper nouns are the official names of people, places, or things. They are always capitalized. Examples include Thomas or San Antonio, Texas. Common nouns are nouns that refer to general types of people, places, or things. Examples include balls, horses, and girls. Abstract nouns refer to qualities or to general ideas. Examples of abstract nouns include democracy and friendship. Collective nouns refer to groups of people, animals, or things. Examples include islands and lambs.

Pronoun

Pronouns take the place of nouns when it is awkward to repeat the same noun several times. A pronoun refers to a word or group of words called an antecedent. Pronouns may be personal or possessive. Personal pronouns refer to specific people, places, or things, and they can be either singular or plural. Possessive pronouns are used to show ownership. Examples of possessive pronouns are his, hers, theirs, and ours. Other types of pronouns include indefinite pronouns (anybody, somebody, everybody), relative pronouns (which, that, who, whoever), and demonstrative pronouns (this, that, these, those).

Possessive personal pronouns

I	My	Mine
He	His	
She	Her	Hers
We	Our	Ours
You	Your	Yours
They	Their	Theirs
It	Its	Its

Adjective

An adjective is a word or phrase that modifies a noun. Adjectives can also modify pronouns. Adjectives are the words that are used to answer the questions: which one, how many, what kind, and how much. Other parts of speech, such as nouns, verbs, and pronouns, can act like adjectives. In the structure of a sentence, the adjective will generally come before the noun or phrase that it modifies. Examples of adjective phrases include a hard test, a shallow pool, a loud speaker, a yellow shoe, and a slow walker.

> ➤ **Review Video: <u>Adjectives</u>**
> *Visit **mometrix.com/academy**
> and enter **Code: 470154***

Verb

A verb expresses an action or state of being. A verb is the word that gives a sentence life. Verbs have tenses, which convey if the action happened in the past, is happening in the present, or will happen in the future. Verb tenses include past, present, and future tenses. Verbs may also come in the form of linking verbs, which do not convey action. They join the subject of a sentence to a pronoun or noun. They are commonly associated with the senses of taste, touch, sight, sound, and smell. For example, tastes, looks, and stinks are some of the sensory linking verbs. Linking verbs include are, am, is, was, were, being, appear, grow, turn, remain, and been.

> ➤ **Review Video: <u>Verbs</u>**
> *Visit **mometrix.com/academy**
> and enter **Code: 743142***

Adverb

Adverbs are words or phrases that modify a verb, adjective, or adverb. Adverbs can be identified because they usually end in the letters ly. They answer the questions how, what, where, and to what degree. Adverbs can be located in various positions throughout a sentence. Adverbs can be conjunctive. Conjunctive adverbs join two clauses together. Examples of conjunctive adverbs include also, likewise, meanwhile, and next. Using a conjunctive adverb usually requires the aid of a semicolon.

> ➤ **Review Video: <u>Adverbs</u>**
> *Visit **mometrix.com/academy**
> and enter **Code: 713951***

Preposition

Prepositions show the relationship of a noun or pronoun to another word in the sentence. A preposition introduces a word or phrase, called the object of the preposition. Prepositions indicate the temporal, spatial, or logical relationships of their objects to the rest of the sentence. Prepositions may occur in the form of prepositional phrases. Prepositional phrases include a preposition, its object, and the associated adjectives or adverbs. These prepositional phrases can act as nouns, adjectives, or adverbs. Examples of prepositions include about, below, during, toward, and under.

> ➤ **Review Video: <u>Prepositions</u>**
> *Visit **mometrix.com/academy**
> and enter **Code: 946763***

Conjunction

Conjunctions are words that can be used to link other words, phrases, and clauses. Conjunctions can be coordinating, subordinating, or correlating. Coordinating conjunctions include the words and, but, or, nor, for, so, and yet. They are used to join words and independent clauses. Correlating conjunctions link equivalent sentence elements, and appear in pairs. Examples of correlating conjunction pairs include both/and, either/or, neither/nor, and so/as.

> ➤ **Review Video: <u>Coordinating and Correlative Conjunctions</u>**
> *Visit **mometrix.com/academy**
> and enter **Code: 390329***

Subordinating conjunctions are used to introduce dependent clauses. Examples include after, although, as, because, how, if, and while.

> ➤ **Review Video:**
> **Subordinating Conjunctions**
> *Visit mometrix.com/academy*
> *and enter Code:* **958913**

Interjection

Interjections are used to express emotions. They can also appear as exclamations. Interjections are not grammatically related to any other word in a sentence. In formal writing, interjections most often appear as part of a direct quotation. Examples of interjections include ouch, yikes, surprise, hey, and stop. All of these words can be used to express a heightened sense of emotion. They convey surprise, anger, excitement, or displeasure.

Prepositions

There are many prepositions in the English language. Some of these are:

aboard
about
above
across
after
against
along
amid
among
around
at
aside
atop
before
behind
below
beneath
beside
between
beyond
but
by
circa
concerning

despite
down
during
except
failing
following
for
from
in
inside
into
like
mid
minus
near
next
of
off
on
onto
opposite
out
outside
over
pace
past
per
plus
regarding
round
save
since
than
through
throughout
times
to
toward
under
underneath
until
up
upon
via
with
within
without

Dependent and independent clauses

Clauses are composed of words that have a distinct subject and predicate. A clause may be independent or dependent. Independent clauses are groups of words that combine to form a complete thought. In other words, an independent clause is a complete sentence. It does not require any other words or phrases to express a complete idea. A dependent clause contains a subject and verb, but it is not a complete thought. It is not a sentence. A dependent clause often contains a word that indicates it is dependent. Some of the words that indicate a dependent clause are after, although, as, because, if, unless, when, and while.

> **Review Video: Clauses**
> *Visit **mometrix.com/academy**
> and enter Code: **893014***

Direct and indirect objects

Direct and indirect objects are both parts of speech within the structure of a sentence. A direct object is the person or thing that is directly affected by the action of the verb. Direct objects answer the questions what or whom. Direct objects can be a single word, a phrase, or a clause. An indirect object is the person or thing that is indirectly affected by the action of the verb. Indirect objects are only used when a direct object is also present. Indirect objects answer the questions to whom, for whom, and for what. In the structure of a sentence, indirect objects are located between the verb and the direct object.

> **Review Video:**
> **Direct and Indirect Objects**
> *Visit **mometrix.com/academy**
> and enter Code: **817385***

Punctuation

Commas

Flow
Commas break the flow of text. To test whether they are necessary, while reading the text to yourself, pause for a moment at each comma. If the pauses seem natural, then the commas are correct. If they are not, then the commas are not correct.

Nonessential clauses and phrases
A comma should be used to set off nonessential clauses and nonessential participial phrases from the rest of the sentence. To determine if a clause is essential, remove it from the sentence. If the removal of the clause would alter the meaning of the sentence, then it is essential. Otherwise, it is nonessential.
Example:

> John Smith, who was a disciple of Andrew Collins, was a noted archeologist.

In the example above, the sentence describes John Smith's fame in archeology. The fact that he was a disciple of Andrew Collins is not necessary to that meaning. Therefore, separating it from the rest of the sentence with commas, is correct.

Do not use a comma if the clause or phrase is essential to the meaning of the sentence.
Example:

> Anyone who appreciates obscure French poetry will enjoy reading the book.

If the phrase "who appreciates obscure French poetry" is removed, the sentence would indicate that anyone would enjoy reading the book, not just those with an appreciation for obscure French poetry. However, the sentence implies that the book's enjoyment may not be for everyone, so the phrase is essential.

Another perhaps easier way to determine if the clause is essential is to see if it has a comma at its beginning or end. Consistent, parallel punctuation must be used, and so if you can determine a comma exists at one side of the clause, then you can be certain that a comma should exist on the opposite side.

Independent clauses
Use a comma before the words and, but, or, nor, for, yet when they join independent clauses. To determine if two clauses are independent, remove the word that joins them. If the two

clauses are capable of being their own sentence by themselves, then they are independent and need a comma between them.
Example:

He ran down the street, and then he ran over the bridge.

He ran down the street. Then he ran over the bridge. These are both clauses capable of being their own sentence. Therefore a comma must be used along with the word "and" to join the two clauses together.

If one or more of the clauses would be a fragment if left alone, then it must be joined to another clause and does not need a comma between them.
Example:

He ran down the street and over the bridge.

He ran down the street. Over the bridge. "Over the bridge" is a sentence fragment and is not capable of existing on its own. No comma is necessary to join it with "He ran down the street".

Note that this does not cover the use of "and" when separating items in a series, such as "red, white, and blue". In these cases a comma is not always necessary between the last two items in the series, but in general it is best to use one.

Parenthetical expressions
Commas should separate parenthetical expressions such as the following: after all, by the way, for example, in fact, on the other hand.
Example:

By the way, she is in my biology class.

If the parenthetical expression is in the middle of the sentence, a comma would be both before and after it.
Example:

She is, after all, in my biology class.

However, these expressions are not always used parenthetically. In these cases, commas are not used. To determine if an expression is parenthetical, see if it would need a pause if you were reading the text. If it does, then it is parenthetical and needs commas.

Example:

You can tell by the way she plays the violin that she enjoys its music.

No pause is necessary in reading that example sentence. Therefore the phrase "by the way" does not need commas around it.

> **Review Video: Commas**
> *Visit* **mometrix.com/academy**
> *and enter* **Code: 644254**

Hyphens
Hyphenate a compound adjective that is directly before the noun it describes.
Example 1:

He was the best-known kid in the school.

Example 2:

The shot came from that grass-covered hill.

Example 3:

The well-drained fields were dry soon after the rain.

Semicolons

Period Replacement
A semicolon is often described as either a weak period or strong comma. Semicolons should separate independent clauses that could stand alone as separate sentences. To test where a semicolon should go, replace it with a period in your mind. If the two independent clauses would seem normal with the period, then the semicolon is in the right place.

Example:

The rain had finally stopped; a few rays of sunshine were pushing their way through the clouds.

The rain had finally stopped. A few rays of sunshine were pushing their way through the clouds. These two sentences can exist independently with a period between them.

Because they are also closely related in thought, a semicolon is a good choice to combine them.

Transitions
When a semicolon is next to a transition word, such as "however", it comes before the word.
Example:
> The man in the red shirt stood next to her; however, he did not know her name.

If these two clauses were separated with a period, the period would go before the word "however" creating the following two sentences: The man in the red shirt stood next to her. However, he did not know her name. The semicolon can function as a weak period and join the two clauses by replacing the period.

> ➤ **Review Video: Transitions**
> *Visit **mometrix.com/academy**
> and enter **Code: 707563***

Test Tips

Usage

Each question includes a sentence with four parts underlined. You must choose which, if any, of those underlined portions contains an error in mechanics, word choice, or structural and grammatical relationships. If there aren't any errors in any of the underlined parts, you can always select "No Error" as your fifth answer choice.

Word Confusion
"Which" should be used to refer to things only.
> John's dog, which was called Max, is large and fierce.

"That" may be used to refer to either persons or things.
> Is this the only book that Louis L'Amour wrote?
> Is Louis L'Amour the author that [or who] wrote Western novels?

"Who" should be used to refer to persons only.
> Mozart was the composer who [or that] wrote those operas.

Correct pronoun usage in combinations
To determine the correct pronoun form in a compound subject, try each subject separately with the verb, adapting the form as necessary. Your ear will tell you which form is correct.
Example:
> Bob and (I, me) will be going.

Restate the sentence twice, using each subject individually. Bob will be going. I will be going. "Me will be going" does not make sense.

When a pronoun is used with a noun immediately following (as in "we boys"), say the sentence without the added noun. Your ear will tell you the correct pronoun form.
Example:
> (We/Us) boys played football last year.

Restate the sentence twice, without the noun. We played football last year. Us played football last year. Clearly "We played football last year" makes more sense.

> ➤ **Review Video: Pronoun Usage**
> *Visit **mometrix.com/academy**
> and enter **Code: 666500***

Sentence Correction

Each question includes a sentence with part or all of it underlined. Your five answer choices will offer different ways to reword or rephrase the underlined portion of the sentence. The first answer choice merely repeats the original underlined text, while the other four offer different wording.

These questions will test your ability of correct and effective expression. Choose your answer carefully, utilizing the standards of written English, including grammar rules, the proper choice of words and of sentence construction. The correct answer will flow smoothly and be both clear and concise.

Use your ear

Read each sentence carefully, inserting the answer choices in the blanks. Don't stop at the first answer choice if you think it is right, but read them all. What may seem like the best choice, at first, may not be after you have had time to read all of the choices. Allow your ear to determine what sounds right. Often one or two answer choices can be immediately ruled out because it doesn't make sound logical or make sense.

Contextual clues

It bears repeating that contextual clues offer a lot of help in determining the best answer. Key words in the sentence will allow you to determine exactly which answer choice is the best replacement text.
Example:

> Archeology has shown that some of the ruins of the ancient city of Babylon are approximately 500 years <u>as old as any supposed</u> Mesopotamian predecessors.
>
> A.) as old as their supposed
> B.) older than their supposed

In this example, the key word "supposed" is used. Archaeology would either confirm that the predecessors to Babylon were more ancient or disprove that supposition. Since supposed was used, it would imply that archaeology had disproved the accepted belief, making Babylon actually older, not as old as, and answer choice "B" correct.

Furthermore, because "500 years" is used, answer choice A can be ruled out. Years are used to show either absolute or relative age. If two objects are as old as each other, no years are necessary to describe that relationship, and it would be sufficient to say, "The ancient city of Babylon is approximately as old as their supposed Mesopotamian predecessors," without using the term "500 years".

> ➢ **Review Video: <u>Context</u>**
> *Visit **mometrix.com/academy**
> and enter **Code: 613660**

Simplicity is bliss

Simplicity cannot be overstated. You should never choose a longer, more complicated, or wordier replacement if a simple one will do. When a point can be made with fewer words, choose that answer. However, never sacrifice the flow of text for simplicity. If an answer is simple, but does not make sense, then it is not correct.

Beware of added phrases that don't add anything of meaning, such as "to be" or "as to them". Often these added phrases will occur just before a colon, which may come before a list of items. However, the colon does not need a lengthy introduction. The phrases "of which [...] are" in the below examples are wordy and unnecessary. They should be removed and the colon placed directly after the words "sport" and "following".

Example 1:

> There are many advantages to running as a sport, *of which the top advantages are*:

Example 2:

> The school supplies necessary were the following, *of which a few are*:

Mathematics Test

The Mathematics Test section of the HESI A^2 exam consists of 50 questions.
All numbers used are real numbers.
Jagged or straight lines can both be assumed to be straight.

50 minutes are allotted for this portion of the exam.

Basic Math

Common Number Groupings

Natural numbers: also called counting numbers; include the natural sequence of numbers you would recite if someone directed you to count from 1 to 10; natural numbers can be any number from 1 to infinity.
Whole numbers: like natural numbers, except they include the number 0.
Odd numbers: all numbers *not* evenly divisible by 2; the set ranges from 1 to infinity
Even numbers: includes all numbers evenly divisible by 2; ranges from 0 to infinity
Rational numbers: any number that can be expressed as a quotient of two integers; includes fractions
Irrational numbers: includes numbers that are generally represented by symbols, such as π, $\sqrt{12}$, and φ
Prime numbers: numbers divisible only by 1 and themselves; includes 3, 7, and 13
Composite numbers: numbers divisible by numbers other than 1 and themselves; they include 2, 6, and 10

Order of Operations

Many mathematical problems will feature several different operations. In order to solve an equation correctly, one must perform the steps in the correct order. The first step is to perform operations contained within parentheses. The second step is to perform any operations that contain roots and powers. Third, perform multiplication and division operations (from left to right). The fourth step is to perform all addition and subtraction operations (from left to right). The order of operations is often recalled with the simple mnemonic "Please Excuse My Dear Aunt Sally": 1. Parentheses, 2. Exponents, 3. Multiplicationand Division (from left to right), 4. Addition and Subtraction (from left to right).

> ➤ **Review Video: Order of Operations**
> Visit *mometrix.com/academy*
> and enter *Code:* **259675**

Rounding Numbers

Rounding a number may seem like a simple task, but, like many mathematical operations, it is governed by a set of rules. First, determine the place value of the number that must be rounded. For example, if you must round 52.7 to the nearest whole number, the number 52 is the number that must be rounded. Next, observe the number to the immediate right of the number that must be rounded. If that number is 5 or greater, add 1 to the number that must be rounded. In the example 52.7, the 7 is greater than 5, so the rounded number will be 53. If the number to the right is 5 or less, the number will remain unchanged. For example, 52.3 would be rounded to 52.

Factors

Factors are whole numbers that can be multiplied together to equal another whole number. For example, 4 multiplied by 5 equals 20. The numbers 4, 5, and 20 are all whole numbers, while the numbers 4 and 5 are factors of 20. Some numbers have only one or two factors, while others have several factors. One type of factor is the common factor. Common factors are the numbers that are factors to two or more whole numbers. When asked to determine the common factors of a series of numbers, first find the factors of each number.

For example, find the common factors of 9, 12, and 15. The factors of 9 are 1, 3, and 9; the factors of 12 are 1, 2, 3, 4, 6, and 12; and the factors of 15 are 1, 3, 5 and 15. The common factors are 1 and 3, because these are the only factors that all three numbers have in common. The greatest common factor is 3 and the least common factor is 1.

> **Review Video: Factors**
> *Visit **mometrix.com/academy** and enter **Code: 920086***

Roman Numerals

Whole number	Roman numeral	Whole number	Roman numeral
1	I	6	VI
2	II	7	VII
3	III	8	VIII
4	IV	9	IX
5	V	10	X

> **Review Video: Convert Arabic Numerals to Roman Numerals**
> *Visit **mometrix.com/academy** and enter **Code: 994275***

> **Review Video: Convert Roman Numerals to Arabic Numerals**
> *Visit **mometrix.com/academy** and enter **Code: 530931***

Solving Algebraic Equations

Variables are letters that represent an unknown number. You must solve for that unknown number in single variable problems. The main thing to remember is that you can do anything to one side of an equation as long as you do it to the other.

Example:
Solve for x in the equation $2x + 3 = 5$.

Answer: First you want to get the "2x" isolated by itself on one side. To do that, first get rid of the 3. Subtract 3 from both sides of the equation $2x + 3 - 3 = 5 - 3$ or $2x = 2$. Now since the x is

being multiplied by the 2 in "2x", you must divide by 2 to get rid of it. So, divide both sides by 2, which gives $2x / 2 = 2 / 2$ or $x = 1$.

Rules for Solving Algebraic Equations

Similar to order of operation rules, algebraic rules must be obeyed to ensure a correct answer. Begin by locating all parentheses and brackets, and then solving the equations within them. Then, perform the operations necessary to remove all parentheses and brackets. Next, convert all fractions into whole numbers and combine common terms on each side of the equation. Beginning on the left side of the expression, solve operations involving multiplication and division. Then, work left to right solving operations involving addition and subtraction. Finally, cross-multiply if necessary to reach the final solution.

Example 1:
$$4a - 10 = 10$$

The variable in this equation is a. Variables are most commonly presented as either x or y, but they can be any letter. Every variable is equal to a number; one must solve the equation to determine what that number is. In an algebraic expression, the answer will usually be the number represented by the variable. In order to solve this equation, keep in mind that what is done to one side must be done to the other side as well. The first step will be to remove 10 from the left side by adding 10 to both sides. This will be expressed as $4a - 10 + 10 = 10 + 10$, which simplifies to $4a = 20$. Next, remove the 4 by dividing both sides by 4. This step will be expressed as $4a \div 4 = 20 \div 4$. The expression now becomes $a = 5$.

Example 2:
$$12 = -4(-6x - 3)$$
$$12 = 24x + 12$$
$$12 - 12 = 24x + 12 - 12$$
$$0 = 24x$$
$$0/24 = x$$
$$\text{thus } x = 0$$

- 35 -

Example 3:

$$-3(4x + 3) + 4(6x + 1) = 43$$
$$-12x + (-9) + 24x + 4 = 43$$
$$12x + (-5) = 43$$
$$12x = 43 + 5$$
$$12x = 48$$
$$x = 48/12$$
$$\text{thus } x = 4$$

Positive/Negative Numbers

A number can be either positive or negative. The signs + and – are used to indicate the positive or negative value of a number, respectively. Positive numbers can be written with or without the plus sign. Negative numbers must always be written with the minus sign. However, it is common practice when working with positive and negative numbers in the same instance to use the signs for both the positive and negative numbers. For example, when creating a chart with a number line, all negative numbers should have the minus sign, and all positive numbers should have the plus sign. This prevents any confusion. The number 0 is the point that separates positive and negative numbers. Looking at a number line, all of the numbers to the left of 0 are negative, and all of the numbers to the right are positive.

Addition/Subtraction

In mathematical equations with both positive and negative numbers, the correct order of operations must be observed or the answer will be incorrect. For addition of numbers with the same sign, simply add the numbers and leave the sign as is. For example: +10 + 9 = +19. For addition of numbers with different signs, begin by subtracting the smaller number from the larger number. To finish the equation, place the sign of the larger number on the final answer. For example, -12 + 8 = -4. In a subtraction operation, there is a number that is being subtracted (the subtrahend) and a number that is being subtracted from (the minuend). The subtrahend will follow the operation sign. In order to subtract numbers that are both positive, both negative, or opposite values, one must first change the sign on the subtrahend to its opposite

value. Then, change the minus operator to a plus sign. Now that you have converted the subtraction problem into an addition problem, complete the problem following the rules for addition as explained above.

Example:
Treat a negative sign just like a subtraction sign.
$$3 + -2 = 3 - 2 \text{ or } 1$$

Example:
Remember that you can reverse the numbers while adding or subtracting.
$$-4 + 2 = 2 + -4 = 2 - 4 = -2$$

Example:
A negative number subtracted from another number is the same as adding a positive number.
$$2 - -1 = 2 + 1 = 3$$

Example:
Beware of making a simple mistake!
An outdoor thermometer drops from 42º to – 8º. By how many degrees has the outside air cooled?

Answer: A common mistake is to say 42º – 8º = 34º, but that is wrong. It is actually 42º - - 8º or 42º + 8º = 50º

> ➤ **Review Video:**
> **Addition and Subtraction**
> *Visit **mometrix.com/academy***
> *and enter **Code: 521157***

Multiplication/Division

When multiplying positive numbers, negative numbers, or numbers with opposite signs, multiply as if all the numbers were positive numbers. In order to determine which sign to place on the final product, count the number of negative signs in the problem. If the number of negative signs is even, the product will be positive. If the number of negative signs is odd, the answer will be negative. However, if there are an equal number of positive and negative signs in the problem, the product will be positive. To divide a series of positive and negative numbers, divide them as if they were all positive. As in multiplication, the number of negative signs will determine the sign for the quotient. An even number of negative signs indicates the quotient will be positive. An odd number of negative signs indicates the quotient will be negative.

Example:
A negative multiplied or divided by a negative = a positive number.

$$-3 * -4 = 12; \quad -6 / -3 = 2$$

Example:
A negative multiplied by a positive = a negative number.

$$-3 * 4 = -12; \quad -6 / 3 = -2$$

> ➤ **Review Video:**
> **Multiplication and Division**
> *Visit **mometrix.com/academy**
> and enter **Code: 643326***

Fractions

A fraction contains a numerator and a denominator. Numerators are the numbers on the top of the fraction, and denominators are on the bottom. Types of fractions include proper, improper, and mixed numbers. A proper fraction has a numerator that is smaller than the denominator. For example, the fractions $\frac{4}{18}$, $\frac{12}{13}$ and $\frac{9}{22}$, are all proper. An improper fraction has a numerator that is larger than or equal to its denominator. For example, $\frac{8}{8}$ and $\frac{15}{6}$ are improper fractions. Mixed numbers are made up of a whole number and a fraction. For example, $2\frac{2}{3}$ and $7\frac{3}{4}$ are mixed numbers. Dividing a fraction is also known as reducing it. A fraction can be reduced by dividing the numerator and denominator by a number that can go into both evenly. For example, $\frac{6}{12}$ can be divided by $\frac{6}{6}$ to reach its lowest term, $\frac{1}{2}$. Multiplying a fraction

is known as raising it. In order to raise a fraction, multiply the numerator and denominator by the same number. For example, $\frac{2}{3}$ multiplied by $\frac{3}{3}$ will produce $\frac{6}{9}$.

> ➤ **Review Video: Fractions**
> *Visit **mometrix.com/academy**
> and enter **Code: 262335***

Improper Fractions, Whole or Mixed Numbers

Improper fractions are those that have a numerator that is greater than the denominator. This indicates that one whole piece is present, with some left over. If the improper fraction is 8/8, it can be converted into the whole number 1. Any fraction that has the same numerator and denominator can be converted into the whole number 1. An improper fraction (such as $\frac{21}{4}$) can be converted by dividing the denominator into the numerator. $\frac{21}{4}$ will become $5\frac{1}{4}$. A fraction such as $\frac{12}{6}$ would simply become the whole number 2. Mixed numbers can also be turned into fractions. Using the example $5\frac{1}{4}$, convert into a fraction by multiplying the denominator and the whole number. This will result in the number 20. Now, add the numerator to this number to get 21. This number will become the numerator while the original denominator remains the same, yielding $\frac{21}{4}$.

> ➤ **Review Video: Proper and Improper**
> **Fractions and Mixed Numbers**
> *Visit **mometrix.com/academy**
> and enter **Code: 211077***

Adding Fractions

Adding fractions requires that all denominators be the same. If this is not the case, steps must be taken to convert all of the denominators. The first step when adding fractions with different denominators is to determine the lowest common denominator. Consider the problem $\frac{3}{4}$ + $\frac{3}{12}$ + $\frac{5}{24}$. The lowest common denominators of 4, 12, and 24 are found by listing the multiples of each number. The multiples of 4 are 4, 8, 12, 16, and 24; the multiples of 12 are 12 and 24; and the multiple of 24 is 24. The number 24 is the smallest number common to all of the denominators. Now each fraction must be changed so that 24 is the denominator. To make $\frac{3}{4}$ a fraction with a denominator of 24, multiply it by $\frac{6}{6}$ (equivalent to 1) to get $\frac{18}{24}$. Multiply $\frac{3}{12}$ by $\frac{2}{2}$ to get $\frac{6}{24}$. The problem thus becomes $\frac{18}{24}$ + $\frac{6}{24}$ + $\frac{5}{24}$. Finally, add all of the numerators together and allow the denominator to remain the same. The answer will be $\frac{29}{24}$ or $1\frac{5}{24}$.

Subtracting Fractions

Subtracting fractions can only be done when all denominators are the same. If this is not the case, the denominators must be converted. Begin by determining the least common denominator of all the fractions. As an example, consider the problem $\frac{2}{7}$ – $\frac{5}{14}$ – $\frac{2}{21}$. To find the least common denominator, begin by listing the multiples of each denominator. Multiples of 7 include 7, 14, 21, 28, 35, and 42; multiples of 14 include 14, 28, and 42; multiples of 21 include 21 and 42. The least common denominator is 42. Next, convert each fraction into one with a denominator of 42. $\frac{2}{7}$ becomes $\frac{12}{42}$, $\frac{5}{14}$ becomes $\frac{15}{42}$, and $\frac{2}{21}$

becomes $\frac{4}{42}$. $\frac{12}{42}$ – $\frac{15}{42}$ – $\frac{4}{42}$ will yield - $\frac{7}{42}$.

This can be reduced to - $\frac{1}{6}$.

> ➢ **Review Video:**
> **Adding and Subtracting Fractions**
> *Visit **mometrix.com/academy**
> and enter **Code: 378080***

Multiplying Fractions

Unlike adding and subtracting fractions, multiplying fractions does not require a shared denominator. Fraction multiplication is achieved by simply multiplying numerators together and then multiplying denominators together. In most cases, the product will be a large fraction that can be reduced. For example, $\frac{5}{12}$ x $\frac{4}{7}$ = $\frac{20}{84}$. This fraction can be reduced to $\frac{5}{21}$. Some problems will be presented as mixed numbers, such as $1\frac{2}{3}$ x $2\frac{3}{4}$ In order to multiply these fractions, first convert the mixed numbers into improper fractions. $1\frac{2}{3}$ becomes $\frac{5}{3}$ and $2\frac{3}{4}$ becomes $\frac{11}{4}$. The problem $\frac{5}{3}$ x $\frac{11}{4}$ will produce $\frac{55}{12}$. This improper fraction can be converted into the mixed number $4\frac{7}{12}$.

> ➢ **Review Video: Multiplying Fractions**
> *Visit **mometrix.com/academy**
> and enter **Code: 638849***

Dividing Fractions

The division of fractions is made possible by converting the problem into a multiplication problem. In order to divide two fractions, first invert the fraction that follows the division operator. Consider $\frac{4}{5}$ ÷ $\frac{3}{4}$. The fraction following

- 38 -

the division operator is $\frac{3}{4}$, so this must be inverted to $\frac{4}{3}$. Now, change the division sign to a multiplication sign. The problem $\frac{4}{5} \div \frac{3}{4}$ becomes $\frac{4}{5} \times \frac{4}{3}$. Following the normal multiplication rules for fractions, simply multiply the numerators together and then multiply the denominators together. The result will be $\frac{16}{15}$. This, of course, is an improper fraction, which can be converted into the mixed number $1\frac{1}{15}$.

> ➤ **Review Video: <u>Dividing Fractions</u>**
> Visit **mometrix.com/academy**
> and enter **Code: 300874**

Decimal and Percents

Places to right of decimal	Name	Example	Fractional equivalent
One	Tenths	0.5	5/10
Two	Hundredths	0.12	12/100
Three	Thousandths	0.227	227/1000
Four	Ten-thousandths	0.2578	2,578/10,000
Five	Hundred-thousandths	0.45261	45,261/100,000
Six	Millionths	0.214556	214,556/1,000,000

Converting Decimals to Fractions

A fraction can be turned into a decimal and vice versa. In order to convert a fraction into a decimal, simply divide the numerator by the denominator. For example, the fraction $\frac{5}{4}$ becomes 1.25. This is done by dividing 5 by 4. The fraction $\frac{4}{8}$ becomes 0.5 when 4 is divided by

8. This remains true even if the fraction $\frac{4}{8}$ is first reduced to $\frac{1}{2}$. The decimal conversion will still be 0.5. In order to convert a decimal into a fraction, count the number of places to the right of the decimal. This will be the number of zeros in the denominator. The numbers to the right of the decimal will become the whole number in the numerator.

Examples:

$0.45 = \frac{45}{100}$

$\frac{45}{100}$ reduces to $\frac{9}{20}$

$0.237 = \frac{237}{1000}$

$0.2121 = \frac{2121}{10000}$

Adding and Subtracting

When adding and subtracting decimals, the decimal points must always be aligned. Adding decimals is just like adding regular whole numbers.

Example:
    4.5 + 2 = 6.5.

If the problem-solver does not properly align the decimal points, an incorrect answer of 4.7 may result. An easy way to add decimals is to align all of the decimal points in a vertical column visually. This will allow one to see exactly where the decimal should be placed in the final answer. Begin adding from right to left. Add each column in turn, making sure to carry the number to the left if a column adds up to more than 9. The same rules apply to the subtraction of decimals.

> ➤ **Review Video: <u>Adding and Subtracting Decimals</u>**
> Visit **mometrix.com/academy**
> and enter **Code: 381101**

Multiplying Decimals

A simple multiplication problem has two components: a multiplicand and a multiplier. When multiplying decimals, work as though the numbers were whole rather than decimals. Once the final product is calculated, count the number of places to the right of the decimal in both the multiplicand and the multiplier. Then, count that number of places from the right of the product and place the decimal in that position. For example, 12.3 x 2.56 has three places to the right of the respective decimals. Multiply 123 x 256 to get 31488. Now, beginning on the right, count three places to the left and insert the decimal. The final product will be 31.488.

> **Review Video: <u>Multiplying Decimals</u>**
> *Visit **mometrix.com/academy***
> *and enter **Code: 731574***

Dividing Decimals

Every division problem has a divisor and a dividend. The dividend is the number that is being divided. In the problem 14 ÷ 7, 14 is the dividend and 7 is the divisor. In a division problem with decimals, the divisor must be converted into a whole number. Begin by moving the decimal in the divisor to the right until a whole number is created. Next, move the decimal in the dividend the same number of spaces to the right. For example, 4.9 into 24.5 would become 49 into 245. The decimal was moved one space to the right to create a whole number in the divisor, and then the same was done for the dividend. Once the whole numbers are created, the problem is carried out normally: 245 ÷ 49 = 5.

> **Review Video: <u>Dividing Decimals</u>**
> *Visit **mometrix.com/academy***
> *and enter **Code: 560690***

Converting Decimals, Fractions, and Percentages

Percentages are a type of fraction. In a percentage, the denominator, represented by a % sign, is always 100. The sign % stands for per hundred. So, 25% can be read as 25 per hundred. In order to convert a decimal to a percent, move the decimal point two spaces to the right. The decimal 0.45 becomes 45%. In order to convert a percentage into a decimal, move the decimal point two places to the left. The percentage 16% becomes 0.16. Fractions can also be converted into percentages. The first step is to convert the fraction into a decimal. Next, convert the decimal into a percentage. For example, consider the fraction $\frac{3}{4}$. Dividing 3 by 4 yields 0.75, which can be converted into a percentage by shifting the decimal two places to the right (75%).

> **Review Video: <u>Converting Decimals to Fractions and Percentages</u>**
> *Visit **mometrix.com/academy***
> *and enter **Code: 986765***

> **Review Video: <u>Converting Fractions to Percentages and Decimals</u>**
> *Visit **mometrix.com/academy***
> *and enter **Code: 306233***

> **Review Video: <u>Converting Percentages to Decimals and Fractions</u>**
> *Visit **mometrix.com/academy***
> *and enter **Code: 287297***

Decimal and Fraction Equivalents

Fraction	Decimal	Percentage
1/4	0.25	25%
1/2	0.50	50%
3/4	0.75	75%
1/3	$0.\overline{3}$ *	$33.\overline{3}$ %
2/3	$0.\overline{6}$ *	$66.\overline{6}$ %
1/5	0.20	20%
3/5	0.60	60%
4/5	0.80	80%
1/6	$0.1\overline{6}$ *	$16.\overline{6}$ %
5/6	$0.8\overline{3}$ *	$83.\overline{3}$ %
1/8	0.125	12.5%
3/8	0.375	37.5%
5/8	0.625	62.5%
7/8	0.875	87.5%

* the symbol $^{-}$ above a number indicates that the number to the right is repeated infinitely.

Percents

Example:
A percent can be converted to a decimal simply by dividing it by 100.
What is 2% of 50?

Answer: 2% = 2/100 or .02, so .02 * 50 = 1

Exponents

Exponents are the numbers that appear in superscript form to the right of a whole number. For example, in 3^6 the 6 is the exponent and 3 is the base number. The exponent indicates the number of times the number should be multiplied by itself. Using the previous example, 3 will be multiplied by itself 6 times (3 x 3 x 3 x 3 x 3 x 3). Base numbers may be either positive or negative. Exponents can be added, subtracted, multiplied, and divided. When performing one of these operations with exponents, simplify each base and then proceed with the mathematical operation. For example, $5^2 + 2^3$ would be solved by figuring out that $5^2 = 25$ and $2^3 = 8$. The problem becomes 25 + 8, which equals 23.

> ➢ **Review Video: Exponents**
> *Visit **mometrix.com/academy**
> and enter **Code: 600998***

Examples:

Whole number	Number squared	Number cubed
0	0	0
1	1	1
2	4	8
3	9	27
4	16	64
5	25	125
6	36	216
7	49	343
8	64	512
9	81	729
10	100	1,000
11	121	1,331
12	144	1,728

Example:
When exponents are multiplied together, the exponents are added to get the final result.
$x*x = x^2$, where x^1 is implied and 1 + 1 = 2.

Example:
When exponents in parentheses have an exponent, the exponents are multiplied to get the final result.
$(x^3)^2 = x^6$, because 3*2 = 6.

Another way to think of this is that $(x^3)^2$ is the same as $(x^3)*(x^3)$. Now you can use the multiplication rule given above and add the exponents, 3 + 3 = 6, so $(x^3)^2 = x^6$

Multiple exponents
In equations where each base has only one exponent, the solution involves first solving (or simplifying) each base and then carrying out the

mathematical operations. However, some equations have base numbers raised to multiple powers. As an example, consider $(5^2)^3$. In order to simplify this base, first multiply the exponents. 2 x 3 = 6, so the base become 5^6, which is equal to 15,625. When multiplying exponents that have the same base number, add the exponents and then simplify. This is only the case when the base numbers are not zero. For example, 2^3 x 2^2 will become 2^5. For division problems where exponents have the same base, subtract the exponents. For example, $2^4 \div 2^2$ is solved by first subtracting 2 from 4. This problem simplifies to $2^2 = 4$.

Decimal Exponents (Scientific Notation)

This usually involves converting back and forth between scientific notation and decimal numbers (e.g. 0.02 is the same as 2×10^{-2}). There's an old "cheat" to this problem: if the number is less than 1, the number of digits behind the decimal point is the same as the exponent that 10 is raised to in scientific notation, except that the exponent is a negative number; if the number is greater than 1, the exponent of 10 is equal to the number of digits ahead of the decimal point minus 1.

> **Review Video: Scientific Notation**
> Visit **mometrix.com/academy**
> and enter **Code: 976454**

Example:
　　　Convert 3000 to decimal notation.

Answer: 3×10^3, since 4 digits are ahead of the decimal, the number is greater than 1, and (4-1) = 3.

Example:
　　　Convert 0.05 to scientific notation.

Answer: 5×10^{-2}, since the five is two places behind the decimal (remember, the exponent is negative for numbers less than 1).

Any number raised to an exponent of zero is always 1. Also, unless you know what you're doing, always convert scientific notation to

"regular" decimal numbers before doing arithmetic, and convert the answer back if necessary to answer the problem.

Mean, Median, and Mode

The most common numbers calculated in statistics are the mean, median, and mode. The mean is also called the average. The mean is calculated by adding a series of numbers together and then dividing that sum by the number of items in the series. Consider the following series: 5, 8, 10, and 13. The sum of these numbers is 36 and there are 4 numbers in the series, so the mean is calculated 36 ÷ 4 = 9. In this example 9 is the mean or average. The median is the number that falls directly in the middle of a series of numbers when they are arranged in ascending or descending order. If a series has an odd number of items, the median is the number in the middle of the series. If the series has an even number of items, the median is the average of the two middle numbers. Using the sequence above, the middle numbers are 8 and 10, the average of which is 9 (8 + 10 =18; 18 ÷ 2 = 9). The mode is the number that appears most often within a series. A series may have no mode, one mode, or multiple modes.

> **Review Video:**
> **Mean, Median, and Mode**
> Visit **mometrix.com/academy**
> and enter **Code: 286207**

Examples:

Series	Mean	Median	Mode
12, 7, 9, 7, 4, 13, 6, 5, 3	$7.\overline{3}$	7	7
54, 34, 62, 17, 45, 9, 12	$33.\overline{285714}$	34	none
2, 4, 6, 8, 10, 12, 14, 17	9.125	9	none
1, 2, 5, 7, 9, 5, 6, 2	4.625	5	2 and 5

Ratios and Proportions

Ratios are numbers that have a relationship to each other. A ratio can be represented as

$a : b$ or $\dfrac{a}{b}$, which are both read as "*a* is to *b*."

➤ **Review Video: Ratios**
*Visit **mometrix.com/academy**
and enter **Code: 996914***

A proportion is two ratios that are equal to each other. For example, $a : b = c : d$ or $\dfrac{a}{b} = \dfrac{c}{d}$. This would be read as "*a* is to *b* as *c* is to *d*." A problem using a proportion may look like this: $\dfrac{a}{10} = \dfrac{5}{20}$. This can be solved by cross-multiplying to get $50 = 20a$. Now divide both sides by 20 to solve for *a*. The final answer is $a = \dfrac{50}{20}$ or $\dfrac{5}{2}$, which can be converted to $2\dfrac{1}{2}$.

➤ **Review Video: Proportions**
*Visit **mometrix.com/academy**
and enter **Code: 505355***

Simple Probability

The probability problems on the HESI A2 exam are fairly straightforward. The basic idea is this: the probability that something will happen is the number of possible ways that something can happen divided by the total number of possible ways for all things that can happen.

➤ **Review Video: Simple Probability**
*Visit **mometrix.com/academy**
and enter **Code: 212374***

Example:
I have 20 balloons, 12 are red, 8 are yellow. I give away one yellow balloon; if the next balloon is randomly picked, what is the probability that it will be yellow?

Answer: The probability is $\dfrac{7}{19}$, because after giving one away, there are 7 different ways that the "something" can happen, divided by 19 remaining possibilities.

Example problem
A swimming pool is filled with floating rubber ducks in four different colors. One third of the ducks are pink, one sixth of the ducks are blue, and one fourth of the ducks are green. The remaining 52 ducks are yellow. How many rubber ducks are in the pool?

$$\text{Total ducks} = x$$
$$\tfrac{1}{3}(x) = \text{pink ducks}$$
$$\tfrac{1}{6}(x) = \text{blue ducks}$$
$$\tfrac{1}{4}(x) = \text{green ducks}$$
$$52 = \text{yellow ducks}$$
$$x = \tfrac{1}{3}(x) + \tfrac{1}{6}(x) + \tfrac{1}{4}(x) + 52$$
$$12x = 4x + 2x + 3x + 624$$
$$12x = 9x + 624$$
$$3x = 624$$
$$x = 208$$

Students must understand how to create a basic equation by assigning only one variable. In this case, the variable *x* is the total number of ducks in the pool. Once the student has solved for *x*, they can go on to calculate the number of each color of duck if necessary. This problem only asks the student to find the total number of rubber ducks in the pool.

Geometry

Other problems may describe a geometric shape, such as a triangle or circle, but may not include a drawing of the shape. The HESI A² exam is testing whether you can read a description and make appropriate inferences by visualizing the object and related information. There is a simple way to overcome this obstacle: DRAW THE SHAPE! A good drawing (or even a bad drawing) is much easier to understand and interpret than a brief description.

Make a quick drawing or sketch of the shape described. Include any angles or lengths provided in the description. Once you can see the shape, you have already partially solved the problem and will be able to determine the right answer.

Formulas for Calculating Area

Shape	Formula for area
Circle	$A = \pi r^2$, where $\pi = 3.14$ and $r =$ radius
Parallelogram	$A = bh$, where $b =$ base and $h =$ height
Rectangle	$A = lw$, where $l =$ length and $w =$ width
Square	$A = s^2$, where $s =$ side
Trapezoid	$A = \frac{1}{2}h(b + a)$, where $h =$ height, $a =$ lower base, and $b =$ upper base
Triangle	$A = \frac{1}{2}bh$, where $b =$ base and $h =$ height

Formulas for Perimeter

Shape	Formula for perimeter
Parallelogram	$P = 2l + 2w$, where $l =$ length and $w =$ width
Rectangle	$P = 2l + 2w$, where $l =$ length and $w =$ width
Square	$P = 4s$, where $s =$ side
Trapezoid	$P = b_1 + b_2 + s_1 + s_2$, where $b_1 =$ lower base, $b_2 =$ upper base, $s_1 =$ one side, and $s_2 =$ opposite side
Triangle	$P = a + b + c$, where a, b, and c are the sides

Other Formulas

Name	Formula
Surface area of a cylinder	$SA = 2(\pi r^2) + h(2\pi r)$, where $r =$ radius and $h =$ height
Surface area of a rectangular solid	$SA = 2lw + 2wh + 2lh$, where $lw =$ area of bottom and top, $wh =$ area of sides, and $lh =$ area of back and front
Surface area of a cube	$SA = s \times s \times 6$, where $s =$ length of a side
Volume of a cylinder	$V = \pi r^2 \times h$, where $\pi = 3.14$, $r =$ radius, and $h =$ height
Volume of a rectangular solid	$V = l \times w \times h$, where $l =$ length, $w =$ width, and $h =$ height
Volume of a cube	$V = s \times s \times s$, where $s =$ length of side
Circumference of a circle	$C = \pi d$, where $\pi = 3.14$ and $d =$ diameter
Distance	$D = rt$, where $r =$ rate and $t =$ time
Percent Change (PC)	$PC =$ amount of change/original cost
Average	Average = sum of n values/N, where $N =$ the total of numbers in the set and $n =$ the value of each number in the set
Probability	$P =$ # successful outcomes/ # possible outcomes
Selling Price	$SP = c + o + p$, where $c =$ cost, $o =$ overhead, and $p =$ profit
Compound Interest* (once per year)	$FV = P(1 + r)$, where $P =$ starting principal and $r =$ rate of return
Compound Interest* (multiple times per year)	$FV = P(1 + r)^{Yn}$, where $P =$ starting principal, $r =$ rate of return, and $Yn =$ # of compounds per year
Simple Interest	$I = P \times R \times T$, where $P =$ principal, $R =$ rate, and $T =$ time

* Compound Interest may also be called Future Value

Pythagorean Theorem

The Pythagorean Theorem was developed by the Greek mathematician and philosopher Pythagoras. He was the founder of the Pythagorean School of Mathematics in Cortona, Italy. The Pythagorean Theorem states that the area of a square built upon the hypotenuse of a right triangle is equal to the sum of the areas of the squares upon the remaining sides. This theorem can be expressed $a^2 + b^2 = c^2$. The variables a and b are the lengths of the sides, while c is the length of the hypotenuse, or the side opposite of the right angle. A right triangle with one side measuring 3 units and another side measuring 4 units must have a third side that measures 5 units. Plugging these numbers into the Pythagorean formula proves these measurements are accurate: $3^2 + 4^2 = 5^2$, or $9 + 16 = 25$.

> ➤ **Review Video: Pythagorean Theorem**
> *Visit **mometrix.com/academy***
> *and enter **Code: 906576***

Lines and Points

Plane geometry is the study of shapes and figures in a two-dimensional plane. Lines and points are two-dimensional entities. In geometry, the characteristics of a line are that it is always straight, it is composed of an indefinite number of points, and it extends indefinitely in one or two directions. Lines may have arrows at one or both ends, indicating the direction in which the line continues. The portion of a line between two specific points is called a line segment. The defining points of a line are the two endpoints. A line is named after its endpoints. If the endpoints are A and F, then the line is called AF. The line name will have a line symbol above it, while the names of line segments will consist only of the letters.

Important Geometric Terms

Rays are lines with one definite terminus. Rays and lines can be combined to create intersecting, perpendicular, and parallel lines.

Intersecting lines are two lines that cross each other at some point.
Perpendicular lines cross each other such that right angles are formed at their intersection.
Parallel lines, unlike perpendicular and intersecting lines, never cross each other. Parallel lines continue in the same direction indefinitely, always remaining exactly the same distance apart and never crossing. Parallel lines may be intersected by a transverse line.

Angles

Single angle types

Angles are part of plane geometry. They exist in a two-dimensional plane that consists of only flat figures. Angles are made up of two rays, lines that have one definite end point and one indefinite end point. An angle is exists when two rays share the same definite end point. The point where the two rays join is called the vertex. Angles can be measured in degrees. There are several single angles, including right, acute, obtuse, and straight. A right angle is exactly 90°, an acute angle measures less than 90°, and an obtuse angle measures greater than 90° but less than 180°. A straight angle measures exactly 180°. A straight angle is actually a line.

> ➤ **Review Video: Angles**
> *Visit **mometrix.com/academy***
> *and enter **Code: 264624***

Multiple angle types

Angles can occur in combination with other angles. Several multiple angle types can occur in a two-dimensional plane. Adjacent angles are one type of multiple angle. An adjacent angle is two angles with one shared ray and the same vertex. Complementary angles are two angles with a combined measurement of exactly 90°. In other words, complementary angles form a right angle. Perpendicular angles are formed by two lines that intersect to form right triangles at their vertex. Supplementary angles can be combined to form a straight line or a 180° angle. Vertical angles are also a type of multiple angle. Vertical angles are formed when two lines intersect to form angles that are not 90°.

Interior and exterior angles

Interior and exterior angles are formed when a transverse line intersects two parallel lines. When this occurs, eight angles are formed. Half of the angles will be inside or between the parallel lines, while the remaining angles will occur above and below the parallel lines. The angles that occur between the parallel lines are called interior angles, while the angles occurring outside the parallel lines are called exterior angles. Interior and exterior angles are a type of multiple angle because they are formed by various lines that share a side and a vertex.

Circles

Unlike a line, a circle does not extend into infinity. A circle has three basic parts. The distance around a circle is known as the circumference, and is represented by the small letter c. The distance from one end of the circle to the other is called the diameter, and is represented by the small letter d. The middle of the circle is called the center, and the distance from the center to the edge is called the radius. The radius, represented by a small letter r, is equal to half of the diameter. When two lines are drawn from the center of a circle to two separate points on the circle's edges, an angle is formed. Many geometry problems will require the student to find the measurement of angles and distances within and around a circle.

Relationships

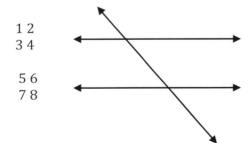

When a transverse line intersects two parallel lines, several things occur. The angles created in 1, 2, 3, and 4 are identical to the angles created in 5, 6, 7, and 8. Specifically, angles 1 and 5, 2 and 6, 3 and 7, and 4 and 8 are equal. These angle pairs are identical, so they are called corresponding angles. Supplementary angles are

formed by 1 and 3, 2 and 4, 1 and 2, 3 and 4, 5 and 7, 6 and 8, 5 and 6, and 7 and 8. Vertical angles are formed by 2 and 3, 1 and 4, 5 and 8, and 6 and 7. A common geometry problem would provide this image and give the measurement of only one angle. The problem would be to find the measurements of the other angles. Because of the various relationships formed when a transverse line intersects parallel lines, it is easy to find all of the angle measurements when given only one measurement.

Triangles

Triangles are three-sided polygons. A triangle consists of three lines and three interior angles. The sum of the angles in a triangle is equal to 180°. The angles inside of a triangle can be acute or obtuse and this determines the type of triangle. Triangles with interior angles that measure less than 90° are called acute triangles. Obtuse triangles have one angle that measures more than 90° but less than 180°. Right triangles have one angle that measures exactly 90°. Triangles may have some sides and angles that are the same, such as in isosceles or equilateral triangles. An isosceles triangle has two equal sides, two equal angles, and one other angle. An equilateral triangle has three equal sides and three equal angles of 60°. Other triangles have no similar pieces, as for instance a scalene triangle, which has no equal sides and no equal angles.

Example problem
> A triangle has three angles. Angle A is 3 times the size of angle B. Angle C is 4 times the size of angle B. Find the measurement of each angle in this triangle.

x = angle B
$3x$ = angle A
$4x$ = angle C
$x + 3x + 4x = 180°$
$8x = 180$
$x = 22.5°$

If $x = 22.5$, then angle B is 22.5°, angle A is 67.5°, and angle C is 90°. Students must know that a

- 46 -

triangle has three angles, whose sum will be 180°. By assigning the variable x to one angle, the student can create an equation that will solve for this variable. Once the value of the variable has been found, the student must remember to solve for all the other angles in the triangle. Answer choices on an actual test may provide a trick answer, where the measurement of only one angle is given. If a student is rushing to finish to test, they may forget to check if the answer they have selected actually matches what the question is asking for. In this question, the answer should include the measurements of all three angles in the triangle.

Squares and Rectangles

A square is a four-sided polygon with sides of equal measure. Each angle inside of a square is exactly 90°, which means the total of all the angles in a square is 360°. By drawing two diagonal lines in a square, connecting the opposite corners, one can form four identical triangles. A common geometry problem may present this drawing and give the measurements of some angles and some sides. The student will have to figure out the remaining measurements. A rectangle is also a four-sided polygon. A rectangle has two long sides and two short sides. The short sides will always be positioned opposite each other. This is also true for the long sides. The interior angles will each be exactly 90°, with a total measurement of 360°. Drawing two diagonal lines inside a rectangle will create two pairs of identical triangles. Students may be asked to find the measurements of all sides and angles when given the measurement of only one side and one angle.

Cubes, Rectangular Solids, and Cylinders

Cubes, rectangular solids, and cylinders are three-dimensional representations of the two-dimensional shapes of squares, rectangles, and circles. Unlike two-dimensional shapes, three-dimensional shapes have the added plane of depth. Two-dimensional figures have area (measured in square inches), while three-dimensional objects have volume (measured in cubic inches). Volume refers to the amount of space inside of an object. Surface area refers to the area on the outside of an object. Students should be familiar with the formulas for calculating the volume and surface area of three-dimensional objects.

> ➤ **Review Video: <u>Volume and Surface Area of a Cube</u>**
> *Visit **mometrix.com/academy** and enter **Code: 664455***

> ➤ **Review Video: <u>Volume and Surface Area of Rectangular Solid</u>**
> *Visit **mometrix.com/academy** and enter **Code: 386780***

Conversion Units

Metric Conversions

1000 mcg (microgram)	1 mg
1000 mg (milligram)	1 g
1000 g (gram)	1 kg
1000 kg (kilogram)	1 metric ton
1000 ml (milliliter)	1 L
1000 L (liter)	1 kl
1000 mm (millimeter)	100 cm
100 cm (centimeter)	10 dm
10 dm (decimeter)	1 m
1 m (meter)	10 dam
10 dam (dekameter)	100 hm
100 hm (hectometer)	1000 km (kilometer)

U.S. and Metric Equivalents

Unit	U.S. equivalent	Metric equivalent
Foot	12 inches	0.305 meters
Yard	3 feet	0.914 meters
Rod	5.5 yards	5.029 meters
Statute mile	1,760 yards	1.609 kilometers
Nautical mile	1,151 statute miles	1.852 kilometers

Area Measurements

Unit	U.S. equivalent	Metric equivalent
Square foot	144 square inches	929.030 square centimeters
Square yard	9 square feet	0.836 square meters
Acre	4,840 square yards	4,072 square meters
section	1 square mile	2,590 square kilometers

Capacity Measurements

Unit	U.S. equivalent	Metric equivalent
Ounce	8 drams	29.573 milliliters
Cup	8 ounces	0.237 liter
Pint	16 ounces	0.473 liter
Quart	2 pints	0.946 liter
Gallon	4 quarts	3.785 liters
Peck	8 quarts	8.810 liters
Bushel	4 pecks	35.239 liters

Weight Measurements

Unit	U.S. equivalent	Metric equivalent
Ounce	16 drams	28.350 grams
Pound	16 ounces	0.45 kg
Ton	2,000 pounds	0.907 metric tons

Units of time

Unit	Equivalent
Minute	60 seconds
Hour	60 minutes
Day	24 hours
Year	365 days
Decade	10 years
Century	100 years
Millennium	1000 years

Nursing Measurements

Unit	English equivalent	Metric equivalent
1 gtt (drop)	1 m (minum)	.06 milliliter
1 tsp	1 fluid dram	5 milliliters
3 tsp	4 fluid drams	15 or 16 milliliters
2 tbsp	1 fluid ounce	30 milliliters
1 glass	8 fluid ounces	240 milliliters
	1 gr (grain)	60 milligrams

Mathematical Symbols

Symbol	Meaning	Example
+	Add	8 + 4
-	Subtract	5 - 3
x or ( ) or ·	Multiply	7 x 5
÷	Divide	14 ÷ 2
=	Equal	5 + 6=11
≠	Not equal	12 ≠ 15
≥	Equal to or greater than	$a \geq b$
≤	Equal to or less than	$a \leq b$
<	Less than	$c < d$
>	Greater than	$c > d$
⊥	Perpendicular to	$f \perp g$
∥	Parallel to	$f \parallel g$
√	Square root	$\sqrt{81}$
³√	Cube root	$\sqrt[3]{18}$
( )	Parentheses	7 (4 + 5)
[ ]	Bracket	6 + [7 (4 + 5)]
{ }	Braces	114 – {6 + [7 (4 + 5)] +2}
∠	Angle	∠ ABC = 25°

Word Problems

Verbal problems are examples of the way that math can be used in everyday life. When a person must increase or decrease a recipe, find the average earnings of their small business, or calculate the amount of chemicals needed to treat their swimming pool, they will not be presented with a nice neat equation. They will have to evaluate the situation and determine which factors are known and which are variables. They will have to decide how to arrange numbers to create the measurements and amounts they need. Standardized tests use word problems to assess a student's ability to apply knowledge of common mathematical skills in a practical situation. Verbal math problems can range from single-step calculations to multiple-step calculations that involve geometry, algebra, and simple arithmetic.

Steps for Solving Word Problems

The first step is to read the problem carefully. Using your own words, summarize the question. Then, identify the known elements of the problem. Identify the variables. Create a picture that will help to visualize the problem. Make a chart or diagram if necessary. Pay attention to the units that are present and consider whether any conversions must be made in order to solve the problem. Analyze the type of information the problem is asking for. Consider whether any formulas apply to the problem. Once you have determined how to solve the problem, perform each mathematical operation carefully. Double check each step for accuracy. Once you have obtained a solution, reconsider the question. Make sure the solution provides a logical and reasonable answer to the question.

Examples

Example 1
　　Heather and Adam are siblings. Heather is 7 years older than Adam. Heather was born in 1987. In what year was Adam born?

x = the year 1987, which is the year of Heather's birth
$x + 7$ = the year Adam was born, because he is 7 years younger than Heather
$1987 + 7 = 1994$

This simple and straightforward problem asks the student to use some basic information to find a specific bit of knowledge. The problem has one basic step—addition. The student must

remember that the question asks for the year Adam was born, not his age.

Example 2
　　Claire and Camille are sisters. Camille is three times as old as Claire. There is exactly 14 years between their ages. How old are Claire and Camille?
x=Claire's age
$3x$=Camille's age
14=difference between Claire and Camille's age
$3x - x = 14$
$2x = 14$
$x = 7$ (Claire's age)
$3x = 21$ (Camille's age)

By assigning a variable to Claire's age, the student can incorporate that same variable into an equation to find the girls' ages. Once the student solves for x, they must remember to perform one more step to solve for Camille's age.

Example 3
　　Two buses leave two different cities located 856 miles apart at the exact same time. Bus A is traveling 65 miles per hour and Bus B is traveling 55 miles per hour. How many hours will it take until the buses meet?

This is a distance problem, and the formula for distance is *distance = rate* x *time* or $d = rt$. In this problem, the question asks for an amount of time. The student must create an expression for the distance each bus travels and then create an equation that uses the information from the problem. The rate of Bus A is 65 mph, and the rate of Bus B is 55 mph. Each rate must be multiplied by the time it will take to travel to a common point, which is unknown. The time is expressed as t. The students must pay careful attention to the units of time used to solve the problem and the units of time required by the question.
　　　$65(t) + 55(t) = 856$
　　　$120(t) = 856$
　　　$t = 7.13$ hours

Example 4

   You are preparing a meal for a social event. If your recipe calls for 3 pounds of ground beef and 5 pounds of lasagna noodles to serve 12, how many pounds will you need to serve 108 people?

This problem is a ratio. Begin by setting up the proportions. Next, cross multiply. Divide by 12 to reach the conclusion that you will need 27 pounds of ground beef to serve 108 people. This problem was created to produce a whole number as an answer, but students should be aware that this is not always the case. Consider if the question is asking you to round up or down. Also, be aware that additional information may be added to the problem to confuse or distract you. You must be able to identify that the amount of pasta needed was irrelevant to this problem.

$$3/12 = x/108$$
$$12x = 324$$
$$x = 27$$

Example 5

   Kevin buys a laptop case on sale. The original price of the case is $60. He paid $27. What was the discount on the case?

Original cost of case = $60
Amount Kevin paid = $27
Difference between original price and sale price = $33
$33/60 = 0.55$ or 55%

Students should be able to complete a basic percent change calculation. In order to find any percent change, the following formula must be used: amount of change ÷ original amount. In this problem, students were given the original amount and the discounted amount. It was necessary to find the difference between the two given amounts in order to complete the calculation.

Example 6

   It costs Grant $30 each to purchase the fishing rods to supply his store. He would like to sell the rods at 50% over the cost. Store overhead runs about $4 for each fishing rod he sells. What is the selling price of each fishing rod?

Cost of fishing rods = $30
Profit = 50% or .50
Overhead = $4
$30 + 4 + (30)(.50) = 49$
Selling price = $49

This problem asks students to use a formula to calculate a selling price. Students must be familiar with the selling price formula, which is selling price = cost = overhead + profit. Profit is calculated by multiplying the cost of an item by the desired profit for the item. Students must also remember that they are looking for a selling price, which will require a dollar sign to precede the answer. Test answer choices for this problem may look like this: A) 49, B) $49, C) $15, D) $17. The correct answer is B because, unlike A, it is expressed in the appropriate units.

Example 7

   The local zoo sold 62 tickets in two hours. Adult admission costs $17.50 and child admission costs $6.25. The zoo made a total of $893.75 in two hours. How many of each type of ticket did the zoo sell?

	Number of tickets	Cost of tickets	Total income
Adult tickets	x	$17.50	$17.50(x)
Child tickets	62-x	$6.25	$6.25(62-x)
Total tickets			$893.75

$$893.75 = 17.50(x) + 6.25(62\text{-}x)$$
$$893.75 = 17.50x + 387.50 - 6.25x$$
$$893.75 = 11.25x + 387.50$$
$$506.25 = 11.25x$$
$$x = 45 \text{ adult tickets and } 62 - 45 = 17 \text{ child tickets}$$

Creating a chart can be very helpful for this kind of problem. Students must understand how total income is calculated in order to solve the problem. Total ticket income = adult ticket income + child ticket income. The problem provides only some of the costs and the total income. Students must understand how to assign a variable (in this case x) to an unknown in order to create an equation.

Example 8
　　Debbie has decided to purchase life insurance. The annual premium rate on $50,000 worth of life insurance is $20 per $10,000. What will Debbie's monthly premium be if she decides to choose this plan?

$20/$10,000 = x/$50,000
$10,000x = $1,000,000
x = $100

The student must set up a proportion equation to determine Debbie's annual premium. Solve for the variable by cross-multiplying. Students must remember that the correct answer will be a dollar amount. Test answer choices may provide the number 100 as a possible choice, but it must have a dollar sign in order to be correct.

Example 9
　　Upon graduation, Ellen's parents give her 500 shares of stock in their family's company. Ellen will receive $13.50 per share in dividend payout each year. How much will Ellen earn in dividends over a three-year period?

$13.50(500) = $6,750
$6,750(3) = $20,250

This problem requires simple multiplication. Students are often confused when faced with problems involving dividends and stocks, because many of them are unfamiliar with this type of scenario. A lack of knowledge about stocks should not interfere with a student's ability to set up a simple equation. Pay close attention to what the problem is asking. The first step reveals the amount of dividends that Ellen receives in one year. The second step reveals

what she will earn in one year. The answer to the problem is $20,250, because that is what Ellen earns over a three-year period. Look out for trick answers, for instance the amount she makes in one year only, or the correct amount absent a dollar sign.

Example 10
　　What is the simple interest on $25,000 invested at 12% annual rate over 2 years?
Principal = $25,000
Rate = 12%
Time = 2 years
x = interest
x = (principal)(rate)(time)
x = ($25,000)(0.12)(2)
x = $6,000

Students must know the formula for calculating simple interest. Students must remember to convert the rate from a percent to a decimal before multiplying. The final answer will be a dollar amount. If the rate were a semiannual rate, students would have to double the amount of the rate (because *semiannual* means twice a year). If the rate were 4.5% semiannually, the annual rate would be 9%.

Example 11
　　Alex uses an Internet sales site to sell baseball cards. Over the last month, he has sold cards for $10, $23, $45, $72, $13 and $22. What is the average price of the cards sold by Alex?

($10 + $23 + $45 + $72 + $13 + $22) ÷ 6 = $30.83

This problem requires students to use a basic statistical formula. An average, or mean, is calculated by finding the sum of all the costs and then dividing by the number of items sold. In this problem, the calculation will result in $30.83, with the final 3 repeating infinitely. A monetary value usually has only two decimal places. In this case, rounding rules require the number to remain at $30.83 because the repeating number is a 3. If the repeating digit had been a 5, students would have to round up to $30.84. Both choices may be provided on a test, to determine

- 51 -

if students understand how to round monetary units.

Example 12

Assume that state tax is 4.75%. Marie purchases a new couch that costs $399.99. What will be the total cost of her purchase once tax is added?

$399.99 + ($399.99)4.75% = total cost
$399.99 + $18.999525 = $418.99

In order to solve this problem, the student must understand the basic equation for calculating the total cost of an item. The student must convert the tax percentage into a decimal before multiplying. 4.75% will become 0.0475. It will produce a very different answer if the student multiplies by 4.75 instead of 0.0475. The student must also remember that the correct answer will contain a dollar sign.

Final Note

As mentioned before, word problems describing shapes should always be drawn out. Remember the old adage that a picture is worth a thousand words. If geometric shapes are described (line segments, circles, squares, etc) draw them out rather than trying to visualize how they should look.

Approach problems systematically; take time to understand what is being asked for. In many cases there is a drawing or graph that you can write on. Draw lines, jot notes, do whatever is necessary to create a visual picture and to allow you to understand what is being asked.

Even if you have always done well in math, you may not succeed on the HESI A^2 exam. While math tests in school will test specific competencies in specific subjects, the HESI A^2 exam frequently tests your ability to apply math concepts from vastly different math subjects in one problem. However, in few cases is any HESI A^2 exam Mathematics Test problem more than two "layers" deep.

What does this mean for you? You can easily learn the HESI A^2 exam Mathematics Test through taking multiple practice tests. If you have some gaps in your math knowledge, we suggest you buy a more basic study guide to help you build a foundation before applying our secrets. Check out our special report to find out which books are worth your time.

Science

Biology

Divisions of Science

The study of science can be divided into physical science and organic science. Physical science is the study of matter and its properties. Physical scientists may study weather patterns, rock composition, or the behavior of energy. Put simply, physical science is the study of nonliving elements. Organic science is the study of living things. Organic scientists seek to understand the forces that allow a living thing to eat, breathe, and reproduce. The divisions of organic science include zoology, biology, and virology. Living things can range from extremely large plants and animals to very tiny cells and viruses.

Entropy and Negentropy

Science often poses the following question: what makes one thing living and another thing non-living? One possible explanation is entropy and negentropy. Entropy refers to the amount of disorder that exists within an object. It can be defined as the tendency of matter to return to a nonliving state. Objects with a relative state of entropy often have a recognizable form (such as a rock or a piece of glass) and are susceptible to the laws of gravity. Objects that do not have entropy are said to have negentropy. Negentropy is a state that requires increasingly large amounts of energy. Objects with negentropy are constantly exchanging matter and undergoing a degree of internal manipulation. In general, objects that have entropy are nonliving, while objects with negentropy are living.

Classification

The classification of living things, in order of increasing specificity: kingdom, phylum, class, order, family, genus, and species. Living things are first classified by kingdom, depending on whether they are plant or animal. Then they are divided into a phylum or subphylum, indicating whether they are vertebrate (with a spinal cord) or invertebrate (without a spinal cord). The next division is known as class. Class can be fish (Pisces), land- and water-dwelling animals (amphibians), birds (avian), reptiles, and mammals. The next division is order, which is exclusive to animals. Order is comprised of meat-eating or vegetable-eating animals. The next division is family, which includes major subdivisions like cat or dog. Next is genus, which is a capitalized Latin name, such as *Homo* for humans. The final division is species, which is a noncapitalized name following the genus.

Five Biological Kingdoms
1. Kingdom animalia: The members of this kingdom are complex, multicellular, eukaryotic organisms that digest food outside their cells and then absorb the digested nutrients. Animals must consume other organisms to obtain most of their nutrients.
2. Kingdom fungi: Kingdom Fungi includes organisms such as slime moulds, mushrooms, smuts, rusts, mildews, moulds, stinkhorns, puffballs, truffles and yeasts. All are classified in this kingdom because they absorb food in solution directly through their cell walls and reproduce through spores. None conduct photosynthesis.
3. Kingdom monera: This is the most primitive of the five kingdoms, it encompasses all the bacteria. Monerans are single-celled prokaryotic organisms.
4. Kingdom plantae: The members of this kingdom are multicellular, eukaryotic organisms that (usually) conduct photosynthesis.
5. Kingdom protista: This kingdom is composed of single-celled (sometimes multicellular), eukaryotic organisms. Protists are more complex than bacteria and include protozooans and some types of algae.

> ➤ **Review Video: Biological**
> **Classification Systems**
> *Visit **mometrix.com/academy***
> *and enter **Code: 736052***

Themes in Biology
Life can be organized into hierarchical levels:
    a. atoms
    b. molecules

c. supramolecular structures

d. cells
- lowest level of organization with all properties of life

e. tissues
- found in some multicellular organisms
- similar cells with specialized functions
- do not display all properties of life

f. organs
- found in some multicellular organisms
- associations of several tissues with an overall specialized function
- do not display all properties of life

g. organisms
- next level with all properties of life
- one or more cells which function together as a reproductive unit

h. populations of organisms

i. communities of different organisms

j. biosphere = totality of all organisms on earth
- some biologists (e.g.: L. Margulis consider populations, communities and even the biosphere, to be "alive")

Biological Organization
Kingdom (one or more phyla)
Phylum (one or more classes)
Class (one or more orders)
Order (one or more classes)
Family (one or more genera)
Genus (one or more species)
Species (a distinct kind or unit)

Three Domains (SuperKingdoms) Of Living Organisms
I. Bacteria: Most of the Known Prokaryotes Kingdom (s): Not Available at This Time Division (Phylum) Proteobacteria: N-Fixing Bacteria Division (Phylum) Cyanobacteria: Blue-Green Bacteria Division (Phylum) Eubacteria: True Gram Positive Bacteria Division (Phylum) Spirochetes: Spiral Bacteria Division (Phylum) Chlamydiae: Intracellular Parasites
II. Archaea: Prokaryotes of Extreme Environments Kingdom Crenarchaeota: Thermophiles Kingdom Euryarchaeota: Methanogens & Halophiles Kingdom Korarchaeota: Some Hot Springs Microbes
III. Eukarya: Eukaryotic Cells Kingdom Protista (Protoctista) Kingdom Fungi Kingdom Plantae Kingdom Animalia

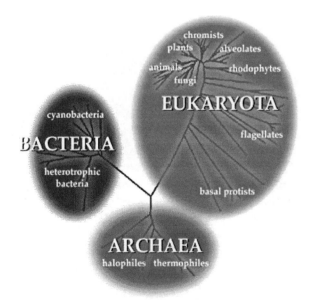

Divisions of simple organisms

Protozoa and bacteria
These simple organisms are capable of producing diseases in humans. These include protozoa, bacteria, fungi, and viruses. Protozoa are single-celled organisms that love moisture. Protozoa are often found in moist areas like the intestines, and may be spread through contaminated water supplies. Bacteria are also single-celled organisms. The human body has a natural balance of good bacteria. When that balance is altered, or when a new bacterium is introduced, the body will become ill. Bacterial infections are the source of cavities, strep throat, and bladder infections. Fungi are multi-celled organisms that are related to plants. These microorganisms invade the body and produce toxins. The toxins result in the symptoms often associated with an illness. For example, toxins may cause sneezing, coughing, fever, and diarrhea.

Fungi and Viruses
There are many microorganisms capable of producing diseases in humans. These include protozoa, bacteria, fungi, and viruses. Fungus can thrive in damp, warm environments, such as the armpits and between the toes. People with compromised immune systems are more susceptible to fungal infections, like athlete's foot and yeast infections. Viruses are dependent upon living cells for the energy they need to thrive. They have a very short life away from living cells. Viruses may be deposited on door knobs and toilet seats. They will die quickly if left exposed. They attach to a host and spread very rapidly, causing serious illness. Viruses are responsible for illnesses such as colds, smallpox, and HIV. These microorganisms invade the body and produce toxins. The toxins cause the symptoms often associated with an illness. For example, toxins may cause sneezing, coughing, fever, and diarrhea.

Cellular Compartments and Organelles

1. Plasma Membrane: All cells are surrounded by a plasma membrane. The plasma membrane is a phospholipid bilayer studded with proteins. Lipids have a hydrophilic head and a hydrophobic tails that, in water, spontaneously form into a bilayer.

Function of the lipids: Keeps the inside in and outside out. Materials enter and exit the membrane through diffusion, osmosis, or membrane transport proteins or recognition proteins.

2. Cytoplasm semifluid "soup" of proteins, enzymes, dissolved salts, sugars. All the organelles and the nucleus float in the cytoplasm.

3. Nucleus contains chromatin: a combination of DNA (genes) and associated proteins, floating in a liquid nucleoplasm, surrounded by nuclear envelope (another lipid bilayer). The nucleolus is an area where synthesis of ribosomal genes rRNA takes place.

4. The EndoMembrane (or CytoMembrane) System:
    A. Ribosomes small structures in the cytoplasm made of RNA and protein that assemble protein chains. Can be "free" in the cytoplasm or bound to the ER
    B. Rough Endoplasmic Reticulum (rough ER) sorts and modifies protein chains delivered by bound ribosomes
    C. Smooth Endoplasmic Reticulum (smooth ER) lacks ribosomes. Site of lipid (membrane) synthesis
    D. Golgi Body connects with the smooth ER, completes lipid synthesis and sorts proteins to their correct destination in small vesicles
    E. Vesicles transport proteins and lipids to the cell surface; bring proteins and lipids into cell from the cell surface, digest compounds (in lysosomes)
    F. Lysosomes: intracellular digestion - contain a potent brew of digestive enzymes
    G. Peroxisomes: break down fatty acids, amino acids, and alcohol

5. Mitochondria: A double membrane-bound organelle that makes ATP for cellular energy (not just one lipid bilayer, but TWO). Contains its own genome.

6. Chloroplast: (Plants only) A double membrane-bound organelle that makes sugar from sunlight and CO_2 during photosynthesis (not just one lipid bilayer, but TWO). Contains its own genome.

7. Cytoskeleton (microtubules and microfilaments) provide cell shape, internal "skeleton" and cell movement.

8. Centioles made of microtubules, may assist in cell division.

9. Cell Wall (Plant, Protists, and Fungi): A tough, rigid (but somewhat elastic) structure made up of cellulose (plants) chitin (fungi) a variety of proteins (protists).

Prokaryotic Cells

<u>Features of Prokaryotic ("pre-nucleus") cells:</u> Few internal parts: bacteria and blue-green algae (Kingdoms Archaebacteria and Eubacteria):

    1. Very small (typically less that 5 microns)
    2. Lack internal compartments and organelles
    3. Lack a nucleus - DNA is not separated from the cytoplasm
    4. One circular chromosome
    5. Tough external walls

> ➤ **Review Video: <u>Eukaryotic and Prokaryotic Cells</u>**
> *Visit **mometrix.com/academy** and enter **Code: 231438***

Eukaryotic Cells

<u>Features of Eukaryotic ('true-nucleus") cells:</u> (Kingdoms: protists, plants, fungi and animals) Numerous internal structures

    1. Subdivided by internal membranes into different compartments
    2. DNA is enclosed by a membrane-bound nucleus
    3. DNA organized into chromosomes

4. Cytoplasm surrounds the nucleus and organelles
5. Plant cells, yeast cells, and protists have a tough cell wall, animal cells do not

Parts of a Cell

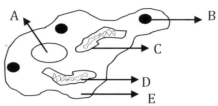

A: Nucleus-largest membrane-bound organelle within a cell; contains the cell's genetic information in the form of DNA; synthesizes RNA, which directs the formation of protein molecules that sustain life; will duplicate itself in order to reproduce
B: Vacuole-energy storage housed within the cytoplasm of a cell; bound by a single-layer membrane; the site of protein and metabolite degradation
C: Cell membrane-acts as a shield to regulate what goes into and comes out of a cell
D: Mitochondria-the powerhouse of the cell; generates energy for the cell through oxidative phosphorylation
E: Cytoplasm-the fluid within the cell membrane; contains the substances that are used by the cell to create energy; consists of 80%-97% water

Diffusion

Living organisms, in order to thrive, must have a process for exchanging gases. In animals, the gases exchanged are oxygen and carbon dioxide. This exchange occurs at a cellular level. Molecules must move through a permeable cell membrane into the cell, where they are converted and then excreted. Diffusion is the process that allows nutrients, gases, and molecules to enter and leave a cell. Diffusion can be facilitated or active. Facilitated diffusion is a form of passive transport that utilizes a transport protein to aide in the diffusion. Passive transport always moves in the direction with the gradient (high to low concentrations). Active transport requires an adenosine triphosphate (ATP) because it moves in the

- 56 -

direction against the gradient (low to high concentrations) and requires a great deal of energy.

➤ **Review Video: <u>Diffusion and Grahams Law of Diffusion</u>**
*Visit **mometrix.com/academy***
*and enter **Code:** 385707*

Osmosis

Osmosis is a type of diffusion. During osmosis, a large molecule is dissolved in water in order to allow it to pass through a cell membrane. Cell membranes are semi-permeable, meaning they only allow some substances to pass through. Consider a starch molecule. Starch molecules are too large to pass through the cell membrane, so they must be dissolved in water. The starch molecules, when they are outside the cell, will interfere with the influx of water into the cell. Water will leave the cell more quickly than it is taken in, allowing the starch to become increasingly diluted. If the starch is inside the cell, water enters the cell more quickly than it leaves, causing the cell to swell. Cells have mechanisms that prevent them from swelling too much, since this could cause a rupture.

Biologic Molecules

Biologic molecules are essential to most living organisms. Carbohydrates are sugars arranged in a long chain. These carbohydrate chains are called polymers. They are essential because they provide structure, energy, and storage. Proteins, the largest of the biologic molecules, are made up of 20 molecules, called amino acids. An enzyme is a type of protein; nearly all cells use enzymes. Nucleic acids are part of the molecules inherited through reproduction. Common nucleic acids are deoxyribonucleic acid (DNA) and ribonucleic acid (RNA).

Lipids as Biologic Molecules
Lipids are more commonly known as fats. They can be fatty acids, phospholipids, or steroids. Fatty acids are either saturated or unsaturated. Unsaturated fats are liquids because they contain one or more double bonds in their hydrocarbon tail. Saturated fats are solid because they contain no double bonds. Phospholipids are made up of two fatty acids bonded to a phosphate group. One end of the phospholipid chain is polar, and the other end is nonpolar. The two ends are attracted to each other, forming a barrier around the cell. Steroids are often components of cellular membranes. They contain a large number of carbon-hydrogen molecules, which makes them nonpolar.

➤ **Review Video: <u>Lipids</u>**
*Visit **mometrix.com/academy***
*and enter **Code:** 269746*

Terminology Review

A
Aerobe. A microorganism that grows in the presence of oxygen.
Amino acid. Any of 20 basic building blocks of proteins- composed of a free amino (NH2) end, a free carboxyl (COOH) end, and a side group (R).
Anaerobe. An organism that grows in the absence of oxygen. See Aerobe.
Antibiotic resistance. The ability of a microorganism to produce a protein that disables an antibiotic or prevents transport of the antibiotic into the cell.
Antibiotic. A class of natural and synthetic compounds that inhibit the growth of or kill other microorganisms. (See Antibiotic resistance, Bacteriocide, Bacteriostat.)
Antibody. An immunoglobulin protein produced by B-lymphocytes of the immune system that binds to a specific antigen molecule. (See monoclonal antibodies, polyclonal antibodies.)
Anticodon. A nucleotide base triplet in a transfer RNA molecule that pairs with a complementary base triplet, or codon, in a messenger RNA molecule. See Codon, Messenger RNA, RNA.
Antigen. Any foreign substance, such as a virus, bacterium, or protein, that elicits an immune response by stimulating the production of antibodies. (See Antigenic determinant, antigenic switching.)
Antigenic determinant. A surface feature of a microorganism or macromolecule, such as a glycoprotein, that elicits an immune response.

Antimicrobial agent. Any chemical or biological agent that harms the growth of microorganisms.

Asexual reproduction. Nonsexual means of reproduction which can include grafting and budding.

Autosome. A chromosome that is not involved in sex de-termination.

B

Bacillus. A rod-shaped bacterium.

Backcross. Crossing an organism with one of its parent organisms.

Bacteriocide. A class of antibiotics that kills bacterial cells.

Bacteriophage (phage or phage particle). A virus that infects bacteria. Altered forms are used as vectors for cloning DNA.

Bacteriostat. A class of antibiotics that prevents growth of bacterial cells.

Bacterium. A single-celled, microscopic prokaryotic organism: a single cell organism without a distinct nucleus.

Base pair (bp). A pair of complementary nitrogenous bases in a DNA molecule--adenine-thymine and guanine-cytosine. Also, the unit of measurement for DNA sequences.

Biologics. Agents, such as vaccines, that give immunity to diseases or harmful biotic stresses.

C

Carcinogen. A substance that induces cancer.

Carcinoma. A malignant tumor derived from epithelial tissue, which forms the skin and outer cell layers of internal organs.

Catalyst. A substance that promotes a chemical reaction by lowering the activation energy of a chemical reaction, but which itself remains unaltered at the end of the reaction.

Catalytic antibody (abzyme). An antibody selected for its ability to catalyze a chemical reaction by binding to and stabilizing the transition state intermediate.

Catalytic RNA (ribozyme). A natural or synthetic RNA molecule that cuts an RNA substrate.

Cation. A positively charged ion.

Centers of origin. Usually the location in the world where the oldest cultivation of a particular crop has been identified.

Centromere. The central portion of the chromosome to which the spindle fibers attach during mitotic and meiotic division.

Chemotherapy. A treatment for cancers that involves ad- ministering chemicals toxic to malignant cells.

Chloramphenicol. An antibiotic that interferes with protein synthesis.

Chromatid. Each of the two daughter strands of a duplicated chromosome joined at the centromere during mitosis and meiosis.

Codon. A group of three nucleotides that specifies addition of one of the 20 amino acids during translation of an mRNA into a polypeptide. Strings of codons form genes and strings of genes form chromosomes. (See Initiation codon, Termination codon.)

Coenzyme (cofactor). An organic molecule, such as a vitamin, that binds to an enzyme and is required for its catalytic activity.

Colony. A group of identical cells (clones) derived from a single progenitor cell.

Conjugation. The joining of two bacteria cells when genetic material is transferred from one bacterium to another.

Cross-hybridization. The hydrogen bonding of a single- stranded DNA sequence that is partially but not entirely complementary to a single-stranded substrate. Often, this involves hybridizing a DNA probe for a specific DNA sequence to the homologous sequences of different species.

Crossing-over. The exchange of DNA sequences between chromatids of homologous chromosomes during meiosis.

Cross-pollination. Fertilization of a plant from a plant with a different genetic makeup.

Culture. A particular kind of organism growing in a laboratory medium.

D

Dalton. A unit of measurement equal to the mass of a hydrogen atom, $1.67 \times 10E-24$ gram/L (Avogadro's number).

Death phase. The final growth phase, during which nutrients have been depleted and cell number decreases. (See Growth phase).

Denature. To induce structural alterations that disrupt the biological activity of a molecule. Often refers to breaking hydrogen bonds between base pairs in double-stranded nucleic acid molecules to produce in single-stranded polynucleotides or altering the secondary and

- 58 -

tertiary structure of a protein, destroying its activity.

Density gradient centrifugation. High-speed centrifugation in which molecules "float" at a point where their density equals that in a gradient of cesium chloride or sucrose. (See Centrifugation.)

Deoxyribonucleic acid. See DNA, nuclease.

Dideoxynucleotide (didN). A deoxynucleotide that lacks a 3' hydroxyl group, and is thus unable to form a 3'-5' phosphodiester bond necessary for chain elongation. Dideoxynucleotides are used in DNA sequencing and the treatment of viral diseases. (See Nucleotide.)

Digest. To cut DNA molecules with one or more restriction endonucleases.

Diploid cell. A cell which contains two copies of each chromosome. See Haploid cell.

DNA (Deoxyribonucleic acid). An organic acid and polymer composed of four nitrogenous bases--adenine, thymine, cytosine, and guanine linked via intervening units of phosphate and the pentose sugar deoxyribose. DNA is the genetic material of most organisms and usually exists as a double-stranded molecule in which two antiparallel strands are held together by hydrogen bonds between adeninethymine and cytosine-guanine. (See b-DNA, cDNA, Complementary DNA or RNA, DNA polymorphism, DNA sequencing, Double-stranded complementary DNA, Duplex DNA, Z-DNA.)

DNA sequencing. Procedures for determining the nucleotide sequence of a DNA fragment.

Dominant gene. A gene whose phenotype is when it is present in a single copy.

Dominant(-acting) oncogene. A gene that stimulates cell proliferation and contributes to oncogenesis when present in a single copy. (See Oncogene.)

Dominant. An allele is said to be dominant if it expresses its phenotype even in the presence of a recessive allele. See Allele, Phenotype, Recessive.

Dormancy. A period in which a plant does not grow, awaiting necessary environmental conditions such as temperature, moisture, nutrient availability.

Double helix. Describes the coiling of the antiparallel strands of the DNA molecule, resembling a spiral staircase in which the paired bases form the steps and the sugar-phosphate backbones form the rails.

Double-stranded complementary DNA (dscDNA). A duplex DNA molecule copied from a cDNA template.

E

Ecology. The study of the interactions of organisms with their environment and with each other.

Ecosystem. The organisms in a plant population and the biotic and abiotic factors which impact on them. See abiotic factors; Biotic factors.

Electrophoresis. The technique of separating charged mol- ecules in a matrix to which is applied an electrical field. (See Agarose gell electrophoresis, Polycrylamide gell electrophoresis.)

Electroporation. A method for transforrning DNA, especially useful for plant cells, in which high voltage pulses of electricity are used to open pores in cell membranes, through which foreign DNA can pass.

Endophyte. An organism that lives inside another.

Enzymes. Proteins that control the various steps in all chemical reactions.

Eukaryote. An organism whose cells possess a nucleus and other membrane-bound vesicles, including all members of the protist, fungi, plant and animal kingdoms; and excluding viruses, bacteria, and blue-green algae. See Prokaryote.

Evolution. The long-term process through which a population of organisms accumulates genetic changes that enable its members to successfully adapt to environmental conditions and to better exploit food resources.

F

FDA. See Food and Drug Administration.

Flanking region. The DNA sequences extending on either side of a specific locus or gene.

Fungus. A microorganism that lacks chlorophyll.

G

Gene insertion. The addition of one or more copies of a normal gene into a defective chromosome.

Gene. A locus on a chromosome that encodes a specific protein or several related proteins. It is considered the functional unit of heredity. (See

Dominant gene, Fusion gene, Gene amplification, Gene expression, Gene flow, Gene pool, Gene splicing, Gene translocation, Recessive gene, Regulatory gene.)

Genetic engineering. The manipulation of an organism's genetic endowment by introducing or eliminating specific genes through modern molecular biology techniques. A broad definition of genetic engineering also includes selective breeding and other means of artificial selection.

Genetic marker. A gene or group of genes used to "mark" or track the action of microbes.

Genotype. The structure of DNA that determines the expression of a trait.

Genus. A category including closely related species. Interbreeding between organisms within the same category can occur.

Growth factor. A serum protein that stimulates cell division when it binds to its cell-surface receptor.

H

Haploid cell. A cell containing only one set, or half the usual (diploid) number, of chromosomes.

Hemophilia. An X-linked recessive genetic disease, caused by a mutation in the gene for clotting factor VIII (hemophilia A) or clotting factor IX (hemophilia B), which leads to abnormal blood clotting.

Homologous chromosomes. Chromosomes that have the same linear arrangement of genes--a pair of matching chromosomes in a diploid organism.

Homologous recombination. The exchange of DNA fragments between two DNA molecules or chromatids of paired chromosomes (during crossing over) at the site of identical nucleotide sequences.

Host. An organism that contains another organism.

Hydrogen bond. A relatively weak bond formed between a hydrogen atom (which is covalently bound to a nitrogen or oxygen atom) and a nitrogen or oxygen with an unshared electron pair.

Hydrolysis. A reaction in which a molecule of water is added at the site of cleavage of a molecule to two products.

I

In situ. Refers to performing assays or manipulations with intact tissues.

In vivo. Refers to biological processes that take place within a living organism or cell.

Incomplete dominance. A condition where a heterozygous off- spring has a phenotype that is distinctly different from, and intermediate to, the parental phenotypes. See Heterozygote, Phenotype.

Insulin. A peptide hormone secreted by the islets of Langerhans of the pancreas that regulates the level of sugar in the blood.

Interferon. A family of small proteins that stimulate viral resistance in cells.

L

Lysis. The destruction of the cell membrane.

M

Malignant. Having the properties of cancerous growth.

Meiosis. The reduction division process by which haploid gametes and spores are formed, consisting of a single duplication of the genetic material followed by two mitotic divisions.

Messenger RNA (mRNA). The class of RNA molecules that copies the genetic information from DNA, in the nucleus, and carries it to ribosomes, in the cytoplasm, where it is translated into protein.

Metabolism. The biochemical processes that sustain a living cell or organism.

Mitosis. The replication of a cell to form two daughter cells with identical sets of chromosomes.

Molecular biology. The study of the biochemical and molecular interactions within living cells.

Mutagen. Any agent or process that can cause mutations. See Mutation.

Mutation. An alteration in DNA structure or sequence of a gene. (See Point mutation.)

N

Natural selection. The differential survival and reproduction of organisms with genetic characteristics that enable them to better utilize environmental resources.

Nucleic acids. The two nucleic acids, deoxyribonucleic acid (DNA) and ribonucleic acid (RNA) are made up of long chains of molecules called nucleotides.

Nucleotide. A building block of DNA and RNA, consisting of a nitrogenous base, a five-carbon sugar, and a phosphate group. Together, the nucleotides form codons, which when strung together form genes, which in turn link to form chromosomes

O

Occupational Safety and Health Administration (OSHA). One of the U.S. agencies responsible for regulation of biotechnology. The major law under which the agency has regulatory powers is the Occupational Safety and Health Act.

Organelle. A cell structure that carries out a specialized function in the life of a cell.

Ovum. A female gamete.

P

Parasitism. The closest association of two or more dissimilar organisms where the association is harmful to at least one.

Pathogen. Organism which can cause disease in another organism.

Persistence. Ability of an organism to remain in a particular setting for a period of time after it is introduced.

Pesticide. A substance that kills harmful organisms (for example, an insecticide or fungicide).

Phenotype. The observable characteristics of an organism, the expression of gene alleles (genotype) as an observable physical or biochemical trait. See Genotype.

Phospholipid. A class of lipid molecules in which a phosphate group is linked to glycerol and two fatty acyl groups. A chief component of biological membranes.

Plaque. A clear spot on a lawn of bacteria or cultured cells where cells have been lysed by viral infection.

Polymer. A molecule composed of repeated subunits.

Polypeptide (protein). A polymer composed of multiple amino acid units linked by peptide bonds.

Polysaccharide. A polymer composed of multiple units of monosaccharide (simple sugar).

Primary cell. A cell or cell line taken directly from a living organism, which is not immortalized.

Prokaryote. A bacterial cell lacking a true nucleus; its DNA is usually in one long strand. See Eukaryote.

Protease. An enzyme that cleaves peptide bonds that link amino acids in protein molecules.

Protein kinase. An enzyme that adds phosphate groups to a protein molecule at serine, threonine, or tyrosine residues.

Protein. A polymer of amino acids linked via peptide bonds and which may be composed of two or more polypeptide chains. (See Polypeptide.)

R

Recessive gene. Characterized as having a phenotype expressed only when both copies of the gene are mutated or missing.

Recombinant DNA. The process of cutting and recombining DNA fragments from different sources as a means to isolate genes or to alter their structure and function.

Recombinant. A cell that results from recombination of genes.

Retrovirus. A member of a class of RNA viruses that utilizes the enzyme reverse transcriptase to reverse copy its genome into a DNA intermediate, which integrates into the hostcell chromosome. Many naturally occurring cancers of vertebrate animals are caused by retroviruses.

Reverse genetics. Using linkage analysis and polymorphic markers to isolate a disease gene in the absence of a known metabolic defect, then using the DNA sequence of the cloned gene to predict the amino acid sequence of its encoded protein.

Ribosomal RNA (rRNA). The RNA component of the ribosome. (See RNA.)

RNA (ribonucleic acid). An organic acid composed of repeating nucleotide units of adenine, guanine, cytosine, and uracil, whose ribose components are linked by phosphodiester bonds. (See Antisense RNA, Heterogeneous nuclear RNA, Messenger RNA, Ribosomal RNA, RNA polymerase, Small nuclear RNA, Transfer RNA.)

S

Sexual reproduction. The process where two cells (gametes) fuse to form one hybrid, fertilized cell. See Asexual reproduction, Gamete, Hybrid.

Subunit vaccine. A vaccine composed of a purified antigenic determinant that is separated from the virulent organism.

Synapsis. The pairing of homologous chromosome pairs during prophase of the first meiotic division, when crossing over occurs.

T

Taq polymerase. A heat-stable DNA polymerase isolated from the bacterium Therrnus aquaticus, used in PCR. (See Polymerase.)

Telomere. The end of a chromosome.

Transcription. The process of creating a complementary RNA copy of DNA.

V

Vaccine. A preparation of dead or weakened pathogen, or of derived antigenic determinants, that is used to induce formation of antibodies or immunity against the pathogen. (See Polyvalent vaccine, Subunit vaccine.)

Vector. An autonomously replicating DNA molecule into which foreign DNA fragments are inserted and then propagated in a host cell. Also living carriers of genetic material (such as pollen) from plant to plant, such as insects.

Virulence. The degree of ability of an organism to cause disease.

Virus. An infectious particle composed of a protein capsule and a nucleic acid core, which is dependent on a host organism for replication. A double-stranded DNA copy of an RNA virus genome that is integrated into the host chromosome during lysogenic infection.

W

Wild type. An organism as found in nature; the organism before it is genetically engineered.

X

X-linked disease. A genetic disease caused by a mutation on the X chromosome. In X-linked recessive conditions, a normal female "carrier" passes on the mutated X chromosome to an affected son.

Chemistry

Molecules

Every substance is made up of several smaller components. The smallest particle of any substance that retains the unique chemical properties of the substance is called a molecule. A molecule is made of two or more atoms held together by a chemical force. Just as atoms make up elements, molecules make up compounds. Consider common table sugar, which is made of carbon, hydrogen, and oxygen. It is grainy and sweet; however, the individual elements of sugar have none of these characteristics. Hydrogen and oxygen are gases, while carbon, which is usually black in color, is a solid at room temperature. Molecules can be formed naturally or synthetically, and there are millions of combinations currently known and yet to be discovered.

> ➤ **Review Video: Molecule**
> Visit **mometrix.com/academy**
> and enter **Code: 349910**

Elements

An element is a substance composed of atoms. Atoms contain an equal number of protons and electrons and therefore do not have an overall charge. Elements are the basic building blocks of all substances, and they cannot be reduced to smaller substances through normal chemical means. An element can only be broken into protons and neutrons when the nucleus of its atoms is bombarded with enough force. Elements usually occur as single atoms, but sometimes they may be diatomic (that is, have two atoms). Some diatomic elements include hydrogen, nitrogen, and oxygen. In rare cases, elements can be triatomic (e.g., ozone) or tetratomic (e.g., phosphorus).

Purpose of elements
Fluorine, Chlorine, Bromide and Iodine are all halogens also known as salt formers. Helium, Neon, Argon, Krypton and Xenon are all inert gases also known as noble gases.

Lithium, Sodium, Potassium, Rubidium, and Cesium are all alkali metals.

Periodic Table

The following periodic table presentation of Chlorine can be broken down into the following:

17-	Atomic number
Cl-	Element symbol
Chlorine-	Element name
34.45-	Atomic Weight

The horizontal rows of the periodic table are called periods. From left to right these are arranged by increasing atomic numbers. The vertical rows have similar chemical similarities. The number of known chemical elements is 109. The periodic table was created by, Dmitri Mendeleev a Russian chemist.

> ➤ **Review Video: Periodic Table**
> Visit **mometrix.com/academy**
> and enter **Code: 154828**

Ions

Ions, in the most basic sense, are electrically charged atoms. The charge can be positive (producing cations) or negative (producing anions). The terms cation and anion arise from what happens when a current is passed through an ionic solution. Two devices are inserted into an ionic solution: an anode and a cathode. Current enters the solution through the anode and leaves through the cathode. When the current is introduced to the ionic solution, positively charged ions will be attracted to the cathode, and negatively charged ions will be attracted to the anode. Ionization is an important part of organic chemistry, because the charge of an ion often determines which other ions it will attract.

Acid-Base Principles

Acid-base is more commonly known as pH. A substance may have an acidic, basic, or neutral pH. A pH of 7 is considered neutral, while anything above 7 is considered basic or alkali, and anything below 7 is considered acidic. Drinking water and bodily fluids are generally neutral. The pH of a substance is a logarithmic measure of the concentration of hydrogen ions present. A logarithmic scale means that there is a ten-fold difference between each successive whole number on the scale. The *p* stands for *potenz* (the potential to be) and the *H* stands for *hydrogen*. In other words, pH is a measure of a substance's potential to become hydrogen.

Atoms

An atom is the simplest unit of an element. Atoms that loose or gain electrons are called ions. Positively charged ions are called cations. Negatively charged ions are called anions. All atoms have a nucleus, which has protons and neutrons present. Protons are positively charged particles found within the nucleus. Neutrons do not carry a charge. The total of neutrons and protons is the mass number. The atomic number is the number of protons found in an atom. One mole of that element is the weight of the element required to equal its atomic weight. A compound is when 2 elements are found together in a definite ratio. The term molecule is a unit of two or more atoms that are bonded together. Avogadro's number 6.02×10^{23} is the number of molecules in one mole of that element.

Atoms can share electrons to bond called a covalent bond, or they can transfer electrons to another atom to form an ionic bond. In addition, a polar bond may be performed between substances in situations that a covalent or ionic bond is not desired. Compounds with various shapes, but the same chemical formula are called isomers.

> ➤ **Review Video: Atoms**
> Visit *mometrix.com/academy*
> and enter *Code:* **905932**

States of Matter

Substances can exist in various states of matter. The three common states of matter are solid, liquid, and gas. Water can exist in all three forms. At O degrees Celsius water is a solid. At 100 degrees Celsius water becomes a gas. In solid form the molecules of water are moving very slowly. In liquid form the molecules of water are moving at a faster pace, and in gas form are highly excited. Converting liquid into a gas is known as evaporation. Converting gas into a liquid is known as condensation. Due to the fact that liquids and gases flow easily they are known as fluids. Transfer of a solid into a gas without going through the liquid state is known as sublimation.

> ➤ **Review Video: States of Matter**
> Visit *mometrix.com/academy*
> and enter *Code:* **742449**

Physical Properties of Water
Water has many unique physical properties. It is the only substance that can be found in nature in all three material states—solid, liquid, and gas. Solid water is ice, and gaseous water is steam. Water must reach a temperature of 32° F in order to freeze and 212° F to boil. On the Celsius scale, the freezing point of water is 0°, and its boiling point is 100°. Water is denser in its liquid state than in its solid state. This is why ice floats. Water also has high degree of surface tension. Water tends to be somewhat elastic. You can observe the elasticity caused by the surface tension of water by dropping powder or a leaf into a cup of water, and observing how they float on the surface.

> ➤ **Review Video: Properties of Water**
> Visit *mometrix.com/academy*
> and enter *Code:* **279526**

Pressure Principles
Gravity exerts a large influence on liquids. Liquids will flow faster when they are allowed to flow downward from a greater distance. This is important for nurses who are infusing patients with intravenous solutions. Human bodies, as well as many man-made medical devices, function by using pressure to move liquids and gases. Liquids and gases have a tendency to flow from areas of high pressure to areas of low pressure. Suction tubes used in operations are an example of how pressure can be applied to manipulate the movement of liquids and gases.

Hydrogen Bonding as it Applies to Water

Hydrogen bonding refers to the cohesion that occurs when a hydrogen atom is attracted to two other atoms, rather than just one. In most cases of hydrogen bonding, there is an attraction between hydrogen and an electronegative oxygen, nitrogen, or fluorineatom. Hydrogen bonds occurring in water involve a hydrogen atom covalently attached to the oxygen atoms of two water molecules. Each water molecule contains a weak partial negative charge in the oxygen atom and a weak partial positive charge in the hydrogen atom. When water molecules are located near each other, the charges in one molecule are attracted to the opposite charges in the other molecule, causing the molecules to bond together. Due to hydrogen bonding, water can remain liquid over a wide range of temperatures.

Heat

Energy taken in or given off during reactions is measured as heat. Heat can be measured in various units. Units include: joule-.239 calories, calorie-degree of energy required to raise one gram of water at 14.5 Celsius degrees by a single degree of Celsius.

Solutions

The concept of solvent and solute are applicable to gases, liquids and solids. A solvent is the host substance and the solute is the substance that is dissolved in the solvent. A solution is a homogeneous mixture of two or more substances. A solution that contains the maximum amount of solute is called a saturated solution. A heterogenous mixture is a solution that contains unequal distribution of solvents in the solution. A physical change is a change in the state of matter. A chemical change is a change in the chemical composition of a compound.

When discussing acid and base relationships. An acid is substance that increases the hydrogen ion concentration in water. A base is a substance that increases the hydroxide ion count in water. A chemical reaction identifies a relationship between reactants and products. Products will be formed during a reaction and identified on the right side of the equation. Catalysts can be used to speed up a reaction or cause a reaction, however they are never destroyed.

> ➢ **Review Video: Solutions**
> *Visit mometrix.com/academy*
> *and enter Code: 995937*

Glossary of Important Terms

A

Absolute zero: The lowest possible temperature (-273.15°C).

Absorption: The process by which a substance is soaked up.

Acid: A substance that can give a proton to another substance. Acids are compounds, containing hydrogen, that can attack and dissolve many substances. Acids are described as weak or strong, dilute or concentrated, mineral or organic. Example: hydrochloric acid (HCl). An acid in water can react with a base to form a salt and water.

Acidic solution: A solution with a pH lower than 7.

Acidity: A general term for the strength of an acid in a solution.

Acid radical: The negative ion left behind when an acid loses a hydrogen ion. Example: Cl- in hydrochloric acid (HCl).

Acid salt: An acid salt contains at least one hydrogen ion and can behave as an acid in chemical reactions. Acid salts are produced under conditions that do not allow complete neutralisation of the acid. For example, sulphuric acid may react with a sodium compound to produce a normal sodium salt, sodium sulphate (Na2SO4), or it may retain some of the hydrogen, in which case it becomes the salt sodium hydrogen sulphate (NaHSO4).

Actinide series or actinide metals. A series of 15 similar radioactive elements between actinium and lawrencium. They are transition metals.

Activated charcoal: A form of carbon, made up of tiny crystals of graphite, which is made by heating organic matter in the absence of air. It is then processed further to increase its pore space and therefore its surface area. Its surface area is about 2000 m2/g. Activated charcoal readily adsorbs many gases and it is therefore widely used as a filter, for example, in gas masks.

Activation energy: The energy required to make a reaction occur. The greater the activation energy of a reaction, the more its reaction rate depends on temperature. The activation energy of a reaction is useful because, if the rate of reaction is known at one temperature (for example, 100°C) then the activation energy can be used to calculate the rate of reaction at another temperature (for example, 400°C) without actually doing the experiment.

Adsorption: The process by which a surface adsorbs a substance. The substances involved are not chemically combined and can be separated. Example: the adsorption properties of activated charcoal.

Alchemy: The traditional 'art' of working with chemicals that prevailed through the Middle Ages. One of the main challenges for alchemists was to make gold from lead. Alchemy faded away as scientific chemistry was developed in the 17th century.

Alcohol: An organic compound which contains a hydroxyl (OH) group. Example: ethanol (CH3CH2OH), also known as ethyl alcohol or grain alcohol.

Alkali/alkaline: A base in (aqueous) solution. Alkalis react with, or neutralise, hydrogen ions in acids and have a ph greater than 7.0 because they contain relatively few hydrogen ions. Example: aqueous sodium hydroxide (naoh).

Alkali metals: A member of Group 1 of the Periodic Table. Example: sodium.

Alkaline cell (or battery): A dry cell in which the electrolyte contains sodium or potassium hydroxide.

Alkaline earth metal: A member of Group 2 of the Periodic Table. Example: calcium.

Alkane: A hydrocarbon with no carbon-to-carbon multiple bonds. Example: ethane, C_2H_6.

Alkene: A hydrocarbon with at least one carbon-to-carbon double bond. Example: ethene, C_2H_4.

Alkyne: A hydrocarbon with at least one carbon-to-carbon triple bond. Example: ethyne, C_2H_2.

Allotropes: Alternative forms of an element that differs in the way the atoms are linked. Example: white and red phosphorus.

Alloy: A mixture of a metal and various other elements. Example: brass is an alloy of copper and zinc.

Amalgam: A liquid alloy of mercury with another metal.

Amorphous: A solid in which the atoms are not arranged regularly (i.e. Glassy). Compare crystalline.

Amphoteric: A metal that will react with both acids and alkalis. Example: aluminium metal.

Anhydrous: Lacking water; water has been removed, for example, by heating. Many hydrated salts are crystalline. (Opposite of anhydrous is hydrous or hydrated.) Example: copper(ii) sulphate can be anhydrous (cuso4) or hydrated (cuso4·5H2O).

Anion: A negatively charged atom or group of atoms. Examples: chloride ion (Cl-), hydroxide ion (OH-).

Anode: The electrode at which oxidation occurs; the negative terminal of a battery or the positive electrode of an electrolysis cell.

Anodising: A process that uses the effect of electrolysis to make a surface corrosion resistant. Example: anodised aluminium.

Antacid: A common name for any compound that reacts with stomach acid to neutralise it. Example: sodium hydrogen carbonate, also known as sodium bicarbonate.

Anti-bumping granules: Small glass or ceramic beads, designed to promote boiling without the development of large gas bubbles.

Antioxidant: A substance that reacts rapidly with radicals thereby preventing oxidation of some other substance.

Aqueous: A solution in which the solvent is water. Usually used as 'aqueous solution'. Example: aqueous solution of sodium hydroxide (naoh(aq)).

Aromatic hydrocarbons: Compounds of carbon that have the benzene ring as part of their structure. Examples: benzene (C_6H_6), naphthalene ($C_{10}H_8$). They are known as aromatic because of the strong pungent smell given off by benzene.

Atmospheric pressure: The pressure exerted by the gases in the air. Units of measurement are kilopascals (kpa), atmospheres (atm), millimetres of mercury (mm Hg) and Torr. Standard atmospheric pressure is 100 kpa, 1atm, 760 mm Hg or 760 Torr.

Atom: The smallest particle of an element; a nucleus and its surrounding electrons.

Atomic mass: The mass of an atom measured in atomic mass units (amu). An atomic mass unit is equal to one-twelfth of the atom of carbon-12. Atomic mass is now more generally used instead of atomic weight. Example: the atomic mass of chlorine is about 35 amu.

Atomic number: Also known as proton number. The number of electrons or the number of protons in an atom. Example: the atomic number of gold is 79 and for carbon it is 4.

Atomic structure: The nucleus and the arrangement of electrons around the nucleus of an atom.

Atomic weight: A common term used to mean the average molar mass of an element. This is the mass per mole of atoms. Example: the atomic weight of chlorine is about 35 g/mol.

B

Base: A substance that can accept a proton from another substance. Example: aqueous ammonia ($NH_3(aq)$). A base can react with an acid in water to form a salt and water.

Basic salt: A salt that contains at least one hydroxide ion. The hydroxide ion can then behave as a base in chemical reactions. Example: the reaction of hydrochloric acid (hcl) with the base, aluminium hydroxide ($Al(OH)_3$) can form two basic salts, $Al(OH)_2Cl$ and $Al(OH)Cl_2$.

Battery: A number of electrochemical cells placed in series.

Bauxite: A hydrated impure oxide of aluminium ($Al_2O_3 \cdot xh_2o$, with the amount of water x being variable). It is the main ore used to obtain aluminium metal. The reddish-brown color of bauxite is mainly caused by the iron oxide impurities it contains.

Blast furnace: A tall furnace charged with a mixture of iron ore, coke and limestone and used for the refining of iron metal. The name comes from the strong blast of air introduced during smelting.

Bleach: A substance that removes color in stains on materials, either by oxidizing or reducing the staining compound. Example: sulphur dioxide (SO_2).

Bond: Chemical bonding is either a transfer or sharing of electrons by two or more atoms. There are a number of types of chemical bond, some very strong (such as covalent and ionic bonds), others weak (such as hydrogen bonds).

Chemical bonds form because the linked molecule is more stable than the unlinked atoms from which it formed. Example: the hydrogen molecule ($H2$) is more stable than single atoms of hydrogen, which is why hydrogen gas is always found as molecules of two hydrogen atoms.

Boyle's Law: At constant temperature, and for a given mass of gas, the volume of the gas (V) is inversely proportional to pressure that builds up (P): P $1/V$.

Brine: A solution of salt (sodium chloride, nacl) in water.

Buffer (solution): A mixture of substances in solution that resists a change in the acidity or alkalinity of the solution when small amounts of an acid or alkali are added.

Burette: A long, graduated glass tube with a tap at one end. A burette is used vertically, with the tap lowermost. Its main use is as a reservoir for a chemical during titration.

C

Capillary: A very small diameter (glass) tube. Capillary tubing has a small enough diameter to allow surface tension effects to retain water within the tube.

Carbohydrate: A compound containing only carbon, hydrogen and oxygen. Carbohydrates have the formula $Cn(H2O)n$, where n is variable. Example: glucose ($C6H12O6$).

Catalyst: A substance that speeds up a chemical reaction, but itself remains unaltered at the end of the reaction. Example: copper in the reaction of hydrochloric acid with zinc.

Catalytic converter: A device incorporated into some exhaust systems. The catalytic converter contains a framework and/or granules with a very large surface area and coated with catalysts that convert the pollutant gases passing over them into harmless products.

Cathode: The electrode at which reduction occurs; the positive terminal of a battery or the negative electrode of an electrolysis cell.

Cation: A positively charged ion. Examples: calcium ion ($Ca2+$), ammonium ion ($NH4+$).

Cell: A vessel containing two electrodes and an electrolyte that can act as an electrical conductor.

Celsius scale (°C): A temperature scale on which the freezing point of water is at 0 degrees and the normal boiling point at standard atmospheric pressure is 100 degrees.

Centrifuge: An instrument for spinning small samples very rapidly. The fast spin causes the components of a mixture that have a different density to separate. This has the same effect as filtration.

Ceramic: A material based on clay minerals which has been heated so that it has chemically hardened.

Change of state: A change between two of the three states of matter, solid, liquid and gas. Example: when water evaporates it changes from a liquid to a gaseous state.

Charles's Law: The volume (V) of a given mass of gas at constant pressure is directly proportional to its absolute temperature (T): V T.

Chromatography: A separation technique using the ability of surfaces to adsorb substances with different strengths. The substances with the least adherence to the surface move faster and leave behind those that adhere more strongly.

Coagulation: A term describing the tendency of small particles to stick together in clumps.

Coherent: Meaning that a substance holds together or sticks together well, and without holes or other defects. Example: Aluminium appears unreactive because, as soon as new metal is exposed to air, it forms a very complete oxide coating, which then stops further reaction occurring.

Combustion: A reaction in which an element or compound is oxidized to release energy. Some combustion reactions are slow, such as the combustion of the sugar we eat to provide our energy. If the combustion results in a flame, it is called burning. A flame occurs where gases combust and release heat and light. At least two gases are therefore required if there is to be a flame. Example: the combustion or burning of methane gas (CH_4) in oxygen gas (O_2) produces carbon dioxide (CO_2) and water (H_2O) and gives out heat and light. Some combustion reactions produce light and heat but do not produce flames. Example: the combustion of carbon in oxygen produces an intense red-white light but no flame.

Compound: A chemical consisting of two or more elements chemically bonded together. Example: Calcium can combine with carbon and oxygen to make calcium carbonate (caco3), a compound of all three elements.

Condensation: The formation of a liquid from a gas. This is a change of state, also called a phase change.

Conduction: (i) the exchange of heat (heat conduction) by contact with another object, or (ii) allowing the flow of electrons (electrical conduction).

Conductivity: The ability of a substance to conduct. The conductivity of a solution depends on there being suitable free ions in the solution. A conducting solution is called an electrolyte. Example: dilute sulphuric acid.

Convection: The exchange of heat energy with the surroundings produced by the flow of a fluid due to being heated or cooled.

Covalent bond: This is the most common form of strong chemical bonding and occurs when two atoms share electrons. Example: oxygen (O_2)

Crystalline: A solid in which the atoms, ions or molecules are organized into an orderly pattern without distinct crystal faces. Examples: copper(ii) sulphate, sodium chloride. Compare amorphous.

Crystallisation: The process in which a solute comes out of solution slowly and forms crystals.

Current: An electric current is produced by a flow of electrons through a conducting solid or ions through a conducting liquid. The rate of supply of this charge is measured in amperes (A).

D

Decay (radioactive decay): The way that a radioactive element changes into another element due to loss of mass through radiation. Example: uranium 238 decays with the loss of an alpha particle to form thorium 234.

Decomposition: The break-down of a substance (for example, by heat or with the aid of a catalyst) into simpler components. In such a chemical reaction only one substance is involved. Example: hydrogen peroxide ($H_2O_2(aq)$) into oxygen ($O_2(g)$) and water ($H_2O(l)$).

Dehydration: The removal of water from a substance by heating it, placing it in a dry atmosphere or using a drying (dehydrating) reagent such as concentrated sulphuric acid.

Density: The mass per unit volume (e.g. G/cm^3).

- 68 -

Desalinization: The removal of all the salts from sea water, by reverse osmosis or heating the water and collecting the distillate. It is a very energy-intensive process.

Detergent: A chemical based on petroleum that removes dirt.

Diffusion: The slow mixing of one substance with another until the two substances are evenly mixed. Mixing occurs because of differences in concentration within the mixture. Diffusion works rapidly with gases, very slowly with liquids.

Dilute acid: An acid whose concentration has been reduced in a large proportion of water.

Disinfectant: A chemical that kills bacteria and other microorganisms.

Displacement reaction: A reaction that occurs because metals differ in their reactivity. If a more reactive metal is placed in a solution of a less reactive metal compound, a reaction occurs in which the more reactive metal displaces the metal ions in the solution. Example: when zinc metal is introduced into a solution of copper(ii) sulphate (which thus contains copper ions), zinc goes into solution as zinc ions, while copper is displaced from the solution and forced to precipitate as metallic copper.

Dissociate: To break bonds apart. In the case of acids, it means to break up, forming hydrogen ions. This is an example of ionization. Strong acids dissociate completely. Weak acids are not completely ionized, and a solution of a weak acid has a relatively low concentration of hydrogen ions.

Dissolve: To break down a substance in a solution without causing a reaction.

Distillation: The process of separating mixtures by condensing the vapors through cooling.

Distilled water: Distilled water is nearly pure water and is produced by distillation of tap water. Distilled water is used in the laboratory in preference to tap water because the distillation process removes many of the impurities in tap water that may influence the chemical reactions for which the water is used.

E

Effervesce: To give off bubbles of gas.

Electrical potential: The energy produced by an electrochemical cell and measured by the voltage or electromotive force (emf).

Electrode: A conductor that forms one terminal of a cell.

Electrolysis: An electrical-chemical process that uses an electric current to cause the break-up of a compound and the movement of metal ions in a solution. The process happens in many natural situations (as for example in rusting) and is also commonly used in industry for purifying (refining) metals or for plating metal objects with a fine, even metal coating.

Electrolyte: An ionic solution that conducts electricity.

Electromotive force (emf): The force set up in an electric circuit by a potential difference.

Electron: A tiny, negatively charged particle that is part of an atom. The flow of electrons through a solid material such as a wire produces an electric current.

Electron configuration: The pattern in which electrons are arranged in shells around the nucleus of an atom. Example: chlorine has the configuration 2, 8, 7.

Element: A substance that cannot be decomposed into simpler substance by chemical means. Examples: calcium, iron, gold.

Emulsion: Tiny droplets of one substance dispersed in another. One common oil in water emulsion is called milk. Because the tiny droplets tend to come together, another stabilizing substance is often needed. Soaps and detergents are such agents, wrapping the particles of grease and oil in a stable coat. Photographic film is an example of a solid emulsion.

Endothermic reaction: A reaction that takes in heat. Example: when ammonium chloride is dissolved in water.

Enzyme: Biological catalysts in the form of proteins in the body that speed up chemical reactions. Every living cell contains hundreds of enzymes that help the processes of life continue.

Ester: Organic compounds formed by the reaction of an alcohol with an acid and which often have a fruity taste. Example: ethyl acetate ($CH_3COOC_2H_5$).

Exothermic reaction: A reaction that gives out substantial amounts of heat. Example: sucrose and concentrated sulphuric acid.

Explosive: A substance which, when a shock is applied to it, decomposes very rapidly, releasing a very large amount of heat and creating a large volume of gases as a shock wave.

F

Fats: Semisolid, energy-rich compounds derived from plants or animals, made of carbon, hydrogen and oxygen. These are examples of esters.

Filtration: The separation of a liquid from a solid using a membrane with small holes (i.e. a filter paper).

Fluid: Able to flow; either a liquid or a gas.

Fluorescent: A substance that gives out visible light when struck by invisible waves, such as ultraviolet rays.

Fraction: A group of similar components of a mixture. Example: In the petroleum industry the light fractions of crude oil are those with the smallest molecules, while the medium and heavy fractions have larger molecules.

Freezing point: The temperature at which a substance undergoes a phase change from a liquid to a solid. It is the same temperature as the melting point.

G

Galvanizing: Applying a thin zinc coating to protect another metal.

Gamma rays: Waves of radiation produced as the nucleus of a radioactive element rearranges itself into a tighter cluster of protons and neutrons. Gamma rays carry enough energy to damage living cells.

Gangue: The unwanted material in an ore.

Gas/gaseous phase: A form of matter in which the molecules form no definite shape and are free to move about to uniformly fill any vessel they are put in. A gas can easily be compressed into a much smaller volume.

Glucose: The most common of the natural sugars ($C_6H_{12}O_6$). It occurs as the polymer known as cellulose, the fiber in plants. Starch is also a form of glucose.

Group: A vertical column in the Periodic Table. There are eight groups in the table. Their numbers correspond to the number of electrons in the outer shell of the atoms in the group. Example: Group 2 contains beryllium, magnesium, calcium, strontium, barium and radium.

H

Half-life: The time it takes for the radiation coming from a sample of a radioactive element to decrease by half.

Halide: A salt of one of the halogens.

Halogen: One of a group of elements including chlorine, bromine, iodine and fluorine in Group 7 of the Periodic Table.

Heat: The energy that is transferred when a substance is at a different temperature to that of its surroundings.

Heat capacity: The ratio of the heat supplied to a substance, compared with the rise in temperature that is produced.

Heat of combustion: The amount of heat given off by a mole of a substance during combustion. This heat is a property of the substance and is the same no matter what kind of combustion is involved. Example: heat of combustion of carbon is 94.05 kcal (x 4.18 = 393.1 kJ).

Hydride: A compound containing just hydrogen and another element, most often a metal. Examples: water (H_2O), methane (CH_4) and phosphine (PH_3).

Hydrous: Hydrated with water.

Hydrogen bond: A type of attractive force that holds one molecule to another. It is one of the weaker forms of intermolecular attractive force. Example: hydrogen bonds occur in water.

I

Incomplete combustion: Combustion in which only some of the reactant or reactants combust, or the products are not those that would be obtained if all the reactions went to completion. It is uncommon for combustion to be complete and incomplete combustion is more frequent. Example: incomplete combustion of carbon in oxygen produces carbon monoxide and not carbon dioxide.

Indicator (acid-base indicator): A substance or mixture of substances used to test the acidity or alkalinity of a substance. An indicator changes color depending on the acidity of the solution being tested. Many indicators are complicated organic substances. Some indicators used in the laboratory include Universal Indicator, litmus, phenolphthalein, methyl orange and bromothymol.

Inorganic substance: A substance that does not contain carbon and hydrogen. Examples: nacl, caco3.

Insoluble: A substance that will not dissolve.

Ion: An atom, or group of atoms, that has gained or lost one or more electrons and so developed an electrical charge. Ions behave differently from electrically neutral atoms and molecules. They can move in an electric field, and they can also bind strongly to solvent molecules such as water. Positively charged ions are called cations; negatively charged ions are called anions. Ions can carry an electrical current through solutions.

Ionic bond: The form of bonding that occurs between two ions when the ions have opposite charges. Example: sodium cations bond with chloride anions to form common salt (nacl) when a salty solution is evaporated. Ionic bonds are strong bonds except in the presence of a solvent.

Ionic compound: A compound that consists of ions. Example: nacl.

Isotope: One of two or more atoms of the same element that have the same number of protons in their nucleus (atomic number), but which have a different number of neutrons (atomic mass). Example: carbon-12 and carbon-14.

L

Latent heat: The amount of heat that is absorbed or released during the process of changing state between gas, liquid or solid. For example, heat is absorbed when a substance melts and it is released again when the substance solidifies.

Liquid/liquid phase: A form of matter that has a fixed volume but no fixed shape.

Litmus: An indicator obtained from lichens. Used as a solution or impregnated into paper (litmus paper), which is dampened before use. Litmus turns red under acid conditions and purple in alkaline conditions. Litmus is a crude indicator when compared with Universal Indicator.

M

Mass: The amount of matter in an object. In everyday use the word weight is often used (somewhat incorrectly) to mean mass.

Matter: Anything that has mass and takes up space.

Melting point: The temperature at which a substance changes state from a solid phase to a liquid phase. It is the same as freezing point.

Meniscus: The curved surface of a liquid that forms in a small bore or capillary tube. The meniscus is convex (bulges upwards) for mercury and is concave (sags downwards) for water.

Metal: A class of elements that is a good conductor of electricity and heat, has a metallic luster, is malleable and ductile, forms cations and has oxides that are bases. Metals are formed as cations held together by a sea of electrons. A metal may also be an alloy of these elements. Example: sodium, calcium, gold.

Mineral: A solid substance made of just one element or compound. Example: calcite is a mineral because it consists only of calcium carbonate; halite is a mineral because it contains only sodium chloride.

Mineral acid: An acid that does not contain carbon and which attacks minerals. Hydrochloric, sulphuric and nitric acids are the main mineral acids.

Mixture: A material that can be separated into two or more substances using physical means. Example: a mixture of copper (ii) sulphate and cadmium sulphide can be separated by filtration.

Molar mass: The mass per mole of atoms of an element. It has the same value and uses the same units as atomic weight. Example: molar mass of chlorine is 35.45 g/mol.

Mole: 1 mole is the amount of a substance which contains Avagadro's number (6×10^{23}) of particles. Example: 1 mole of carbon-12 weighs exactly 12 g.

Molecule: A group of two or more atoms held together by chemical bonds. Example: O2.

N

Neutralisation: The reaction of acids and bases to produce a salt and water. The reaction causes hydrogen from the acid and hydroxide from the base to be changed to water. Example: hydrochloric acid reacts with, and neutralizes, sodium hydroxide to form the salt sodium chloride (common salt) and water. The term is more generally used for any reaction in which the ph changes toward 7.0, which is the ph of a neutral solution.

Neutron: A particle inside the nucleus of an atom that is neutral and has no charge.

Newton (N): The unit of force required to give one kilogram an acceleration of one meter per second every second (1 ms-2).

Nitrate: A compound that includes nitrogen and oxygen and contains more oxygen than a nitrite. Nitrate ions have the chemical formula NO3-. Examples: sodium nitrate nano3 and lead nitrate Pb(NO3)2.

Nitrite: A compound that includes nitrogen and oxygen and contains less oxygen than a nitrate. Nitrite ions have the chemical formula NO2-. Example: sodium nitrite nano2.

Noble gases: The members of Group 8 of the Periodic Table: helium, neon, argon, krypton, xenon, and radon. These gases are almost entirely unreactive.

Noble metals: Silver, gold, platinum and mercury. These are the least reactive metals.

Normal salt: Salts that do not contain a hydroxide (OH-) ion, which would make them basic salts, or a hydrogen ion, which would make them acid salts. Example: sodium chloride (nacl).

Nucleus: The small, positively charged particle at the centre of an atom. The nucleus is responsible for most of the mass of an atom.

O

Organic acid: An acid containing carbon and hydrogen. Example: methanoic (formic) acid (HCOOH).

Organic compound (organic substance; organic material): A compound (or substance) that contains carbon and usually hydrogen. (The carbonates are usually excluded.) Examples: methane (CH4), chloromethane (CH3Cl), ethene (C2H4), ethanol (C2H5OH), ethanoic acid (C2H3OOH), etc.

Organic solvent: An organic substance that will dissolve other substances. Example: carbon tetrachloride (ccl4).

Osmosis: A process whereby molecules of a liquid solvent move through a semipermeable membrane from a region of low concentration of a solute to a region with a high concentration of a solute.

Oxidation: Combination with oxygen or a reaction in which an atom, ion or molecule loses electrons to an oxidising agent. (Note that an

oxidising agent does not have to contain oxygen.) The opposite of oxidation is reduction.

Oxidation number (oxidation state): The effective charge on an atom in a compound. An increase in oxidation number corresponds to oxidation, and a decrease to reduction. Shown in Roman numerals. Example: manganate(iv).

Oxidation-reduction reaction (redox reaction): Reaction in which oxidation and reduction occurs; a reaction in which electrons are transferred. Example: copper and oxygen react to produce copper(ii) oxide. The copper is oxidized, and oxygen is reduced.

Oxide: A compound that includes oxygen and one other element. Example: copper oxide (cuo).

Oxidize: To combine with or gain oxygen or to react such that an atom, ion or molecule loses electrons to an oxidising agent.

Oxidising agent: A substance that removes electrons from another substance being oxidized (and therefore is itself reduced) in a redox reaction. Example: chlorine (Cl2).

P

Period: A row in the Periodic Table.

Periodic Table: A chart organizing elements by atomic number and chemical properties into groups and periods.

Ph: A measure of the hydrogen ion concentration in a liquid. Neutral is ph 7.0; numbers greater than this are alkaline; smaller numbers are acidic.

Phase: A particular state of matter. A substance may exist as a solid, liquid or gas and may change between these phases with addition or removal of energy. Examples: ice, liquid and vapor are the three phases of water. Ice undergoes a phase change to water when heat energy is added.

Photon: A parcel of light energy.

Photosynthesis: The process by which plants use the energy of the Sun to make the compounds they need for life. In six molecules of carbon dioxide from the air combine with six molecules of water, forming one molecule of glucose (sugar) and releasing six molecules of oxygen back into the atmosphere.

Polar solvent: A solvent in which the atoms have partial electric charges. Example: water.

Polymer: A compound that is made of long chains by combining molecules (called monomers) as repeating units. ('Poly' means many, 'mer' means part.) Examples: polytetrafluoroethene or Teflon from tetrafluoroethene, Terylene from terephthalic acid and ethane-1, 2-diol (ethylene glycol).

Pressure: The force per unit area measured in pascals.

Product: A substance produced by a chemical reaction. Example: when the reactants copper and oxygen react, they produce the product, copper oxide.

Proton: A positively charged particle in the nucleus of an atom that balances out the charge of the surrounding electrons.

Proton number: This is the modern expression for atomic number.

Purify: To remove all impurities from a mixture, perhaps by precipitation, or filtration.

Q

Quantitative: Measurement of the amounts of constituents of a substance, for example by mass or volume.

R

Radiation: The exchange of energy with the surroundings through the transmission of waves or particles of energy. Radiation is a form of energy transfer that can happen through space; no intervening medium is required (as would be the case for conduction and convection).

Reactant: A starting material that takes part in, and undergoes, change during a chemical reaction. Example: hydrochloric acid and calcium carbonate are reactants; the reaction produces the products calcium chloride, carbon dioxide and water.

Reaction: The recombination of two substances using parts of each substance to produce new substances. Example: the reactants sodium chloride and sulphuric acid react and recombine to form the products sodium sulphate, chlorine and water.

Reagent: A commonly available substance (reactant) used to create a reaction. Reagents are the chemicals normally kept on chemistry laboratory benches. Many substances called reagents are most commonly used for test purposes.

Redox reaction (oxidation-reduction reaction): A reaction that involves oxidation and reduction; a reactions in which electrons are transferred.

Reducing agent: A substance that gives electrons to another substance being reduced (and therefore itself being oxidized) in a redox reaction. Example: hydrogen sulphide (H_2S).

Reduction: The removal of oxygen from, or the addition of hydrogen to, a compound. Also a reaction in which an atom, ion or molecule gains electrons from a reducing agent. (The opposite of reduction is oxidation.)

Relative atomic mass: In the past, a measure of the mass of an atom on a scale relative to the mass of an atom of hydrogen (mass =1),. Nowadays, a measure of the mass of an atom relative to the mass of one twelfth of an atom of carbon-12. If the relative atomic mass is given as a rounded figure, it is called an approximate relative atomic mass. Examples: chlorine 35, calcium 40, gold 197.

S

Salt: A compound, often involving a metal that is the reaction product of an acid and a base, or of two elements. (Note 'salt' is also the common word for sodium chloride, common salt or table salt.) Example: sodium chloride (nacl) and potassium sulphate (K_2SO_4)

Saponification: A reaction between a fat and a base that produces a soap.

Saturated solution: A solution that holds the maximum possible amount of dissolved material. When saturated, the rate of dissolving solid and that of recrystallisation solid are the same, and a condition of equilibrium is reached. The amount of material in solution varies with the temperature; cold solutions can hold less dissolved solid material than hot solutions. Gases are more soluble in cold liquids than in hot liquids.

Separating column: Used in chromatography. A tall glass tube containing a porous disc near the base and filled with a substance (for example, aluminium oxide, which is known as a stationary phase) that can adsorb materials on its surface. When a mixture is passed through the column, fractions are retarded by differing amounts, so that each fraction is washed through the column in sequence.

Solid/solid phase: A rigid form of matter which maintains its shape, whatever its container.

Solubility: A measure of the maximum amount of a substance that can be contained in a solvent.

Soluble: Readily dissolvable in a solvent.

Solute: A substance that has dissolved. Example: sodium chloride in water.

Solution: A mixture of a liquid (the solvent) and at least one other substance of lesser abundance (the solute). Mixtures can be separated by physical means, for example, by evaporation and cooling.

Solvent: The main substance in a solution.

Anatomy and Physiology

Tissues and Cells

Aerobic and Anaerobic Metabolism

The process of metabolism allows cells to produce the energy essential for survival. Cells can metabolize aerobically or anaerobically.

Aerobic metabolism occurs when there is a rich supply of oxygen. The cell pulls nutrients from carbohydrates, fats, and proteins, and turns the nutrients into energy. Aerobic metabolism is the method most often used, and preferred, by human bodies.

Anaerobic metabolism occurs when there is a shortage of oxygen. It most often occurs as a back-up mechanism. Cells must constantly take in nutrients and produce energy in order to survive. Under normal conditions, the human body takes in enough oxygen to facilitate aerobic metabolism. At certain points, when oxygen is not readily available, cells must rely on anaerobic metabolism in order to survive. Anaerobic metabolism is only meant to be used for short periods. For example, a swimmer who holds his breath for long periods is not taking in much oxygen, so his cells must metabolize anaerobically.

Byproducts of Metabolism
Cells are constantly metabolizing fats, carbohydrates, and proteins in order to produce energy.

During aerobic metabolism, cells produce water and carbon dioxide. The water is used by the body or excreted in urine, while carbon dioxide is excreted during exhalation.

Anaerobic metabolism creates byproducts that are more difficult for the body to handle. When skeletal muscle cells are forced to metabolize anaerobically, they produce lactic acid. Lactic acid can overwhelm the body's buffering and excretion mechanisms and cause muscle cramps, rapid breathing, and vomiting.

Cell Activities

Cells have specialized components, each of which performs an essential function. Cells need a permeable cell membrane in order to absorb nutrients. Animal cells take in oxygen, while plant cells take in carbon dioxide. The cell must have the ability to form complex substances using only simple substances and then excrete the by-products of its metabolic processes. This type of synthesis creates and releases energy. As a result of these processes, the cell has a degree of self-regulation involving temperature and pH balance. Cells are also capable of movement: whole (external) and within itself (internal). Finally, a cell must have the ability to reproduce or duplicate itself.

Static and Dynamic Equilibrium
There are two types of equilibrium: static and dynamic. Static equilibrium occurs when things are at a standstill. Water in a bucket is in a state of static equilibrium because it is not going anywhere. Dynamic equilibrium occurs when two opposing reactions occur at the same rate. Making a hole in the bottom of the bucket will cause the water to rush out of the hole, but if water is poured into the bucket at the same rate that water is leaving through the hole, the system is in dynamic equilibrium. Systems that lack equilibrium undergo the process of diffusion. Molecules will enter and exit a cell membrane through the process of diffusion. The molecules move from areas of high pressure to areas of low pressure.

> ➤ **Review Video: Dynamic Equilibrium**
> *Visit **mometrix.com/academy***
> *and enter **Code: 580793***

Krebs Cycle

The Krebs cycle is a series of reactions that occur within the mitochondria of a cell. The Krebs cycle is sometimes called the citric acid cycle or tricarboxylic acid cycle. The first product generated in the sequence of reactions within the Krebs cycle is citric acid, hence the name the citric acid cycle. The reactions use acetyl units to produce phosphate compounds, which provide energy for the cell. Acetate molecules are oxidized to form two molecules of carbon dioxide and eight atoms of hydrogen. The carbon dioxide is removed from the cell by the blood, while the hydrogen is used for oxidative phosphorylation. The reaction is exothermic and produces one molecule of ATP (adenosine triphosphate) during each cycle. The Krebs cycle is actually the second of three stages in the carbohydrate catabolism process.

Blood

The central tissue of the bone, known as bone marrow, is the source of blood generation. Blood cells are generated primarily in the sternum, iliac crests, and femurs. There are three types of blood cells: red cells, white cells, and platelets. The blood cells are not differentiated until they enter the bloodstream. The cells enter the liquid portion of the bloodstream, which is called plasma. Each type of cell performs a different function. Red blood cells are responsible for transporting hemoglobin to the lungs, where it binds with oxygen. White blood cells fight infectious microorganisms that enter the body. Usually, a person with an infection will have an elevated white blood cell count. Platelets are responsible for slowing blood flow through clotting.

Blood is made up of approximately 45% hematocrit, and 55% plasma. Plasma is primarily water, however contains approximately 7% protein and 1.5 other substances. The proteins found in plasma are: albumin, globulin and fibrinogen. Hematocrit is composed mostly of red blood cells, but also white blood cells and platelets. Platelets can be key in blood clotting to form a plug.

Epithelial Tissue

Tissues are groups of cells with a similar purpose that cluster together. Epithelial tissue, often called skin, is composed of cells that cover the entire external surface of the body. Epithelial tissue also lines internal body parts, such as the GI tract, urinary system, and blood vessels. There are various types of epithelial cells, including squamous, columnar, and ciliated. Ciliated tissue contains microscopic hairs (called cilia) that are used to transport fluids and particles. The esophagus is lined with ciliated epithelial tissue so that mucus can be transported out of the body. When someone coughs, phlegm is produced and carried up the esophagus by cilia. Squamous cells are usually flat in appearance. Columnar cells resemble columns, having a tall, elongated shape.

Connective Tissue

Connective tissue is the substance that makes up bones, cartilage, reticular fibers, collagenous fibers, and fatty tissue. Connective tissue gives an organism shape. In sea animals, the connective tissue often creates a shell to protect the delicate organism. In humans, the connective tissue creates a shell that surrounds and protects vital organs. The chest cavity, backbone, and cranium are all connective tissues that protect the underlying soft organs, like the heart, lungs, spinal cord, and brain. Connective tissue tends to be very strong while maintaining a degree of elasticity. It is responsible for the cohesiveness of the body, providing structure and protection but allowing movement at the same time.

Reproductive Tissue

The reproductive tissue of an organism contains genetic coding. Reproductive tissue is unique in that it will only separate when the correct genetic coding is present. The genetic coding contribution from a male is the sperm, while the genetic coding from a female is an egg. Females are born with a finite number of eggs to be released for fertilization at appropriate times. Sperm is produced just prior to being used. When the egg and sperm combine, they create a new human. The cells begin to divide and turn into the various types of tissues that will eventually form a human body. The tissues continue to develop for nine months within the female's uterus. The baby that is formed will be born fully developed, with its own reproductive tissues.

Muscle Tissue

Muscle tissue is a necessity for most animals and humans, because it makes movement possible. Muscle tissue is sometimes attached to bone and sometimes part of an internal organ system. Muscles must contract and relax in order to facilitate locomotion. Muscle tissue can be smooth, cardiac, voluntary, or involuntary. Smooth muscle tissue is a type of involuntary tissue. It moves substances through the digestive tract. It is also found in blood vessels, which transport blood. Cardiac tissue is exclusively involved with the activities of the heart. Voluntary muscle tissue is attached to bones, where it can control fine and gross motor skills.

Nerve Tissue

Nerve tissue is the most complex tissue in the body. It is very resistant to new growth. Nerve tissue acts as the body's control system, translating a desire to act into the actual physical movement. The nerve tissue receives information about the external environment from various sensory receptors, like the eyes and ears. Nerve tissue is also responsible for regulating the internal workings of the body through the endocrine system. It is capable of maintaining body temperature and directing blood flow. Nerve tissue is either peripheral or central and either sensory or motor.

Cardiorespiratory System

The cardiorespiratory system is responsible for removing unessential substances from cells. It consists of the heart, blood vessels, lungs, and airways. These systems work together to transport oxygen to the muscles and organs and to remove carbon dioxide. Air enters the cardiorespiratory system through the nose and mouth. It travels down the trachea into the right and left bronchus. The bronchus becomes numerous bronchi, each of which terminates in a bronchiole. The bronchioles become alveoli, which resemble popcorn. As air flows into the body, it contacts the lining of the passageways, allowing for diffusion across cell membranes.

Cardiovascular System

The cardiovascular system is vital for providing oxygen and nutrients to tissues and removing waste. The heart is divided into four chambers-two atria and two ventricles-that communicate through orifices on each side. The right atrium receives blood from the venous system and then lets blood fall down into the right ventricle. Blood then goes to the lungs for a new supply of oxygen. Then the blood comes back from the lungs and goes to the left atrium. It then falls into the left ventricle and is pumped into the general circulation. The heart is composed of three layers: epicardium, myocardium and an endocardium. Heart sounds are due to the vibrations produced by blood and valve movements. Blood pressure is the force exerted by blood against the insides of the blood vessels. Heart rate is determined by physical activity, body temperature, and concentration of ions. The heart is controlled by impulses from the S-A node which passes to the A-V node.

The arterial system is responsible for delivering oxygen to various tissues and the venous system is responsible for removing waste and returning blood to the heart.

Hypertension is characterized by elevated arterial pressure and is one of the more common diseases of the cardiovascular system. Arteriosclerosis is accompanied by decreased elasticity of the arterial walls and followed by narrowing of the lumen. Hormones can also play a large role in blood pressure regulation. The hormone *aldosterone* can promote retention of water in the kidneys and increased blood volume, which in turn increases blood pressure.

Key Terms
Tachycardia: abnormally fast heartbeat
Bradycardia: abnormally slow heartbeat
Fibrillation: rapid heart beats
Red blood cell (erythrocyte): transports carbon dioxide and oxygen
White blood cell (leukocyte): fight infection including neutrophils, eosinophils, and basophils

Respiratory System

The respiratory stem includes the nose, nasal cavity, sinuses, pharynx, larynx, trachea, bronchial tree, and lungs. Air enters the nose, travels through the nasal cavity where the air is warmed. The air goes through the pharynx, which functions as a common duct for air and food. Then the larynx, which is at the top of the trachea and holds the vocal cords, allows passage of air. The trachea divides into the right and left bronchi on the way into the bronchial tree and the lungs.

The right lung has three lobes and the left lung has two lobes. Gas exchange occurs between the air and the blood within the alveoli, which are tiny air sacs. Diffusion is the mechanism by which oxygen and carbon dioxide are exchanged.

Breathing is controlled by the medulla oblongata and pons. Inspiration is controlled by changes in the thoracic cavity. Air fills the lung because of atmospheric pressure pushing air in. Expansion of the lungs is aided by surface tension, which holds pleural membranes together. In addition, the diaphragm, which is located just below the lungs and stimulated by phrenic nerve, acts as a suction pump to encourage inspiration. Expiration comes from the recoil of tissues and the surface tension of the alveoli.

Aerobic respiration occurs in the presence of oxygen and mostly takes place in the mitochondria of a cell. Anaerobic respiration occurs in the absence of oxygen and takes place in the cytoplasm of a cell. Both of these mechanisms occur in cellular respiration in humans. With anaerobic respiration glucose is broken down and produces less ATP when compared to aerobic respiration.

Key Terms

Anoxia: absence of oxygen in tissue
Atelectasis: collapse of a lung
Dyspnea: difficulty in the breathing cycle
Hypercapnia: excessive carbon dioxide in the blood
Tidal Volume: amount of air that normally moves in and out of the lungs

Nervous System

The nervous system is made of the central nervous system (CNS) and the peripheral nervous system (PNS). The central nervous system is made up of the brain and the spinal cord. The peripheral nervous system consists of cranial and spinal nerves that innervate organs, muscles and sensory systems. The brain controls: thought, reasoning, memory, sight, and judgment. The brain is made up of four lobes: frontal, parietal, temporal, and occipital. The spinal cord is a made up of neural tracts that conduct information to and from the brain.

Cranial nerves in the peripheral nervous system connect the brain to the head, neck and trunk. Peripheral nerves allow control of muscle groups in the upper and lower extremities and sensory stimulation. The peripheral nerves are spinal nerves that branch off the spinal cord going toward organs and muscles.

The autonomic nervous system controls reflexive functions of the brain. Including "fight or flight" response and maintaining homeostasis. Homeostasis is a state of equilibrium within tissues. The autonomic nervous system uses neurotransmitters to help conduct nerve signals and turn on/off various cell groups.

Nervous tissue is composed of neurons, which are the functional unit of the nervous system. A neuron includes a cell body, and organelles usually found in cells. Dendrites provide receptive information to the neuron and a single axon carries the information away.

Key Terms

Synapse: junction between two neurons
Action potential: threshold at which neurons fire

> ➤ **Review Video: Nervous System**
> *Visit **mometrix.com/academy***
> *and enter **Code: 708428***

Afferent and Efferent Nerves

The nerves within the nervous system can be categorized as either efferent or afferent. Afferent nerves are those that carry impulses from one part of the body to the spinal cord and brain. They enable the body to recognize and respond to external stimuli, such as touch, sight, and sound. Because of their connection to the senses, afferent nerves are also called sensory nerves. Efferent nerves carry impulses from the central nervous system to the internal organs or periphery of the body. These nerves direct movement of the whole body or parts of the body. Efferent nerves are also called motor nerves.

Central Nervous System

The central nervous system (CNS) consists of the spinal cord and the brain. The spinal cord transports sensory information from the peripheral nervous system to the brain. It also transports motor information from the brain to the skeletal muscles, cardiac muscles, smooth muscles, and glands. The brain receives the sensory and motor input from the spinal cord and from its own nerves. One of the main functions of the brain is to process sensory input and coordinate the appropriate motor output. The brain and spinal cord are made up of gray matter and white matter. Gray matter consists of masses of cell bodies and dendrites, covered with synapses. White matter consists of bundles of axons coated with myelin. In the spinal cord, white matter is external to gray matter; in the brain, gray matter is external to white matter.

Peripheral Nervous System

The peripheral nervous system (PNS) includes all of the nerves that run through the body, with the exception of the brain and spinal cord. The peripheral nervous system is broken into somatic and autonomic divisions. The PNS connects the CNS to the rest of the body. Neural signals are transmitted to and from the CNS via the pathways of the PNS. The PNS has two types of neurons: sensory neurons and motor neurons. Sensory neurons are connected to sensory receptors like eyes, ears, and skin. Motor neurons carry signals to and from glands and organs.

Somatic vs. Autonomic Divisions

The peripheral nervous system (PNS) contains the nerve structure located in the limbs and internal organs of the body. The PNS has two divisions: somatic and autonomic. The somatic division transmits nerve impulses to and from the skeletal muscles. When a human or animal decides to move, the somatic division of the PNS is activated. The somatic nervous system allows the body to move when willed to do so. The autonomic division consists primarily of involuntary nerves. These nerves control the internal organs. It functions while an organism is awake and asleep. The actions of the autonomic division of the PNS do not require intention on the part of the organism.

Sympathetic and Parasympathetic Systems

The autonomic division of the peripheral nervous system is further divided into the sympathetic and parasympathetic systems.

The sympathetic nervous system is often referred to as the fight-or-flight mechanism. In other words, this system activates in times of extreme stress or danger, telling the organism whether it should fight or run away. Chemicals are released that temporarily heighten the organism's senses. The sympathetic system originates in the thoracic and lumbar regions of the spinal cord. When activated, the sympathetic system can reduce digestive secretions, increase heart rate, and contract blood vessels.

The parasympathetic nervous system is the active system under normal circumstances. It yields to the sympathetic system in times of crisis, but quickly resumes control once the crisis has passed. This system originates in the brain stem and lower spinal cord. The parasympathetic system counteracts the sympathetic system by slowing the heart rate, constricting the pupils, dilating the blood vessels, and stimulating digestive secretions.

Neuroendocrine System

Thalamus and Hypothalamus

The neuroendocrine system is ruled by the thalamus and hypothalamus, both of which are close to the pituitary gland. There is a thalamus on each side of the brain. The thalamus is a cluster of neurons, consisting of a set of tightly packed nuclei. The sensory pathways from receptors like the eyes, ears, and skin all pass through the thalamus, at which point they are dispersed throughout the cerebral cortex. A hypothalamus is located just below and in front of each thalamus. The hypothalamus acts upon the pituitary gland to regulate blood vessels and glands. It influences emotions, sexual behavior, appetite, and sleep cycles. The hypothalamus receives sensory information primarily from taste and smell receptors.

Pituitary Gland

The pituitary gland regulates all the other glands in the body. It is divided into anterior and posterior regions. The posterior pituitary is responsible for maintaining fluid levels within the body through the secretion of antidiuretic hormones and for stimulating uterine contractions during the birthing process. The anterior pituitary is essential for survival. It regulates the secretion of hormones by other organs, such as cortisone secreted from the kidneys. It also produces growth hormone, which regulates the physical growth of the body and all its parts. The anterior pituitary also secretes a hormone that stimulates the thyroid and aids in metabolism. Additionally, it controls the reproductive functions in both sexes and stimulates milk production in females.

Digestive System

Digestion is the process that food is absorbed. The mouth begins to prepare food for digestion. Teeth grind food into smaller substrates. Then salivary glands, which secrete saliva, begin digestion of the food using enzymes. The pharynx and esophagus allow passage of the food into the stomach. The stomach uses gastric juices and absorbs a small amount of the food. Then, the food goes to the small intestine. The pancreas and the liver release enzymes and bile respectively into the small intestine to aid in absorption. The small intestine is composed of the duodenum, jejunum, and ileum. Then substrates are passed into the large intestine, which has little digestive function. Absorption of water and electrolytes does occur in the large intestine.

Peristalsis is the wave like movement occurring in the digestive system that propels food downward. The alimentary canal is the path food travels from the mouth to the anus. Feces are composed mostly of water and substrates and are not absorbed.

Key Terms
Cholelithiasis: stones in the gallbladder
Diverticulitis: inflammation of the small pouches in the colon, if present
Hepatitis: inflammation of the liver
Stomatitis: inflammation of the mouth
Dyspepsia: indigestion
Enteritis: inflammation of the intestine

Reproductive System

Male reproductive organs are specialized for the formation of sperm (gamete) and transporting sperm. The vas deferens is the tube that sperm travels through. Semen is composed of sperm cells and secretions of the prostate and bulbourethral glands. Semen activates sperm cells. Testosterone is the most important male hormone. Testosterone encourages the development of male sex organs. It is responsible for the development of male secondary sexual characteristics.

Female reproductive organs are specialized for childbirth and development of a fetus. The primary structures are the ovaries, uterus, and vagina. The ovaries release an egg cell (gamete) into the uterus. The product of fertilization is a zygote with 46 chromosomes.
The uterus sustains life for the embryo until childbirth. The vagina allows transportation of the fetus during delivery.

Estrogen and progesterone are the primary female sex hormones. Estrogen is responsible for female sexual characteristics. Progesterone is responsible for changes in the uterus. Low estrogen levels and changes in the female reproductive organs are the result of menopause.

Key Terms
Amenorrhea: absence of menstrual flow
Gestation: 40 weeks of pregnancy
Orchitis: inflammation of a testis
Cesarean section: birth of a fetus through an abdominal incision

Gastrointestinal System

The main function of the gastrointestinal system is to process nutrients and distribute them at the cellular level. This system digests food and then rids the body of waste products. The organs that are included in the gut of the gastrointestinal system are the mouth, pharynx, esophagus, stomach, intestines, small intestines, duodenum, jejunum, ileum, large intestine, cecum, colon, rectum, and anus. This list conveys the order in which food substances pass through the gut, entering the body through the mouth and finally exiting the body through the anus. Other organs that are part of the gastrointestinal system, but not part of the gut, include the liver, gallbladder, pancreas, salivary glands, lips, teeth, tongue, epiglottis, thyroid, and parathyroids. While food does not pass through these organs directly, they aid in digestion.

Urinary System

The urinary system consists of the kidneys, ureters, bladder, and urethra. The kidney functions to remove metabolic wastes from the blood and excrete them. The kidney also helps regulate blood pressure, pH of the blood, and red blood cell production. The basic functional unit of the kidney is the nephron. The nephron consists of a renal corpuscle and a renal tubule. Urine is the end product of the urinary system. The kidneys are involved in filtration, re-absorption and secretion. Glomerular filtration is regulated by osmotic pressure. The ureter is a tube that connects the kidneys and the bladder. Kidney stones can become lodged in the ureter. Peristaltic waves in the ureter force urine to the bladder. The bladder stores urine and forces urine into the urethra. Muscle fibers in the wall of the bladder form the detrusor muscle.

Key Terms
Enuresis: uncontrolled urination
Diuretic: a substance that encourages urination
Pyuria: pus in the urine
Ureteritis: inflammation of the ureter

Musculoskeletal System

Members of the animal kingdom possess a musculoskeletal system, which enables them to move around and interact with their environments. Obviously, movement is crucial because it enables animals to move around to find food, mates, and acceptable living conditions, and to flee from threats. The musculoskeletal system is composed of bone, muscle, joints, bursa, ligaments, and tendons. They each have an independent function but are dependent upon each other to execute those functions.

Integumentary System

Skin is the basis of the integumentary system. The skin protects the inner parts of the body and provides shape. Skin helps the body maintain its temperature, contain fluids, and shield the body from infection. The three layers of the skin are the epidermis, dermis, and subcutaneous tissue. When the body has an excess of certain substances, they are excreted through the skin in sweat. Other components of the integumentary system include hair, nails, sweat glands, and sebaceous glands. Hair helps to maintain body temperature and filter out harmful particles.

> ➤ **Review Video: <u>Functions of the Integumentary System</u>**
> *Visit **mometrix.com/academy** and enter **Code: 398674***

Ear

The external ear collects sound and passes the sound to the tympanic membrane. Then the middle ear increases the force of the sound waves using the malleus, stapes, and incus. Auditory tubes connect the middle ear to throat and help maintain proper pressure. The inner ear consists of complex system of tubes and chambers-osseous, membranous labyrinths and also the cochlea. Auditory impulses are interpreted in the temporal lobes.

Eye

The wall of the eye has an outer, middle and inner layer. The sclera (outer layer) is protective. The cornea refracts light entering the eye and is found on the anterior aspect of the sclera. The choroid coat (middle layer) helps keep the inside of the eye dark. The retina (inner layer) contains the receptor cells. The visual receptors are rods and cones. Rods are responsible for colorless vision in dim light, and cones are responsible for color vision.

Key Terms
Otitis media: inflammation of the middle ear
Diplopia: double vision
Tinnitus: ringing in the ears
Vertigo: sensation of dizziness

➢ **Review Video: The Eye**
Visit **mometrix.com/academy**
and enter **Code: 329071**

Genetics

Genetics is the study of how traits are handed down from one generation to another during reproduction. The study of genetics began with Gregor Mendel, a monk who was given the task of studying inherited traits among garden peas. By cross-breeding varieties of peas, Mendel discovered how traits are passed from generation to generation. Mendel's studies produced evidence of dominant and recessive genes, which behave according to the law of segregation. Mendel discovered that the characteristics of an individual are controlled by genes and that genes occur in pairs. Mendel's research was not recognized until the 1900s.

Heredity and Reproduction

In humans, there are exactly 46 chromosomes. The entire genetic code within a single human contains thousands of gene sequences, which are arranged in chromosomes. They are present in the same number in all cells, except for germ cells (sperm and eggs). Germ cells each contain 23 chromosomes rather than 23 pairs, of which the final chromosomal pair is contributed at the time of fertilization. Males have an X and a Y chromosome, while females have two X chromosomes. The male and female of most land-dwelling species are distinguishable from one another. This differentiation also allows for attraction between the sexes, resulting in reproduction.

Professional Practice

Practice settings

Nurses can work in a variety of industries. The obvious locations where nurses can apply their skills are hospitals, clinics, and doctor's offices. Nurses also practice in community agencies, schools, businesses, military units, summer camps, vacation resorts, and cruise ships. Some nurses put their skills and knowledge to use by teaching others to become nurses in college courses or nursing schools. Nurses can work in nursing homes, retirement communities, ambulatory care agencies, volunteer organizations, private practices, hospices, occupational health facilities, and federal or state agencies.

Nurses' Roles

One of the most basic tasks that a nurse can perform is patient care. Nurses must constantly manage and care for patients. While caring for patients, nurses may perform many other roles, and sometimes they may fill multiple roles at once. Nurses can find themselves in the role of caregiver, comforter, teacher, counselor, role model, protector, advocate, decision maker, case manager, researcher, or communicator. Additionally, it is important to note that nurses do not work exclusively one-on-one with patients; nurses can actually work with groups of patients. In some cases, a nurse will work with a whole family or an entire community.

Career opportunities

A nursing degree will allow you to pursue a variety of career options within the field. In general, the career opportunities for nurses increase as the education level of the nurse increases. In other words, more education can result in better job opportunities and higher pay. In addition to working as a general duty or staff nurse, a nurse may work as a private practice nurse, home health nurse, midwife, or anesthetist. Nurses can focus their careers on teaching others by becoming educators in nursing programs. They can work as clinical specialists, administrators, practitioners, or consultants. Nurses can also focus their career in the area of research. Nurses can actually pursue career paths that target their own special areas of interest. For example, midwives can visit expectant mothers and help them prepare for childbirth in the comfort of their own home.

Qualities of Successful Nurses

Successful nurses possess certain qualities that help them excel at their jobs. A good nurse is a team player. Nurses should be able to work well with their peers. The best nurses are honest, dependable, responsible, and accountable. They are capable of following directions and managing stressful situations. Nurses must understand that they are responsible for the wellbeing of others, and they should avoid abusing substances that could alter their decision-making ability. In other words, nurses should avoid drugs and alcohol. Nurses must be able to care for all patients, regardless of gender, race, religion, or other individual characteristics. Nurses must also be able to control their temper. Patients can be disagreeable and colleagues can be frustrating, but nurses must manage their emotions to perform their job effectively.

Nursing Technicians vs. Generalists

There are three types of programs that nursing candidates can choose to pursue: diploma programs, associate degree programs, and baccalaureate programs. Students who complete diploma programs or associate degree programs are considered technicians. These types of programs prepare students for the technical practice of nursing. In other words, these nurses will focus almost exclusively on patient care. Graduates of nursing baccalaureate programs are considered generalists. These nurses are equipped to work in a variety of health care environments. Nurses with a baccalaureate degree can fill many roles, including (but not limited to) care givers, educators, and consultants. While technicians care for individual patients in a structured setting, a generalist may care for groups of patients in unstructured settings.

Graduate Education Options

Nurses who hold either a master's degree or doctoral degree will have more professional opportunity, as well as higher paying careers. The first step for nurses who wish to pursue higher education in nursing is to obtain a baccalaureate degree. Obtaining a master's degree prepares a nurse to become an educator in various nursing programs. A master's degree also allows a nurse to become a researcher, manager, nurse practitioner, or administrator. Doctoral training allows a nurse to earn degrees in education, nursing science, nursing, and philosophy. A nurse with a doctoral degree can become an educator in undergraduate or graduate nursing programs. He or she can become an advanced clinical researcher, consultant, or independent practitioner.

Nursing Programs

In the United States, there are three types of programs available for those who want to become a registered nurse. Each program has a unique curriculum, accreditation agency, and professional organization. The three programs are associate degree programs, diploma programs, and baccalaureate degree programs. Associate degree programs are the shortest—usually taking only two years to complete. Diploma programs, which take three years to complete, are generally affiliated with a hospital. Baccalaureate programs are the longest type of nursing program, lasting four years. These programs are typically offered at a college or university.

Admissions Departments

Nursing programs consider many factors when deciding which candidates will be accepted. In general, nursing programs will consider a candidate's GPA, SAT or ACT scores, writing ability, community service, interviews, references, and entrance exam scores. Nursing schools must often set high standards for admission because of the number of students attempting to join the program. Each program can only accept a certain number of students, making it a highly competitive field. High GPAs and test scores are all key factors in the selection process; they indicate that a candidate is studious and dedicated, and will do well in rigorous nursing courses. Candidates should also be able to provide a list of references—usually people to whom they are not related. References should be people with whom the candidates have worked, such as teachers and employers.

Financial Requirements

In addition to the time commitment required when entering a nursing program, there is a large financial investment involved. Baccalaureate programs are more expensive than other programs because they take longer to complete. Each student must decide how he or she will pay for his or her nursing education. Working while in school is an option, but nursing courses require many hours outside of the classroom. If obtaining financial aid is an option, students are advised to pursue it. Nursing school costs, in addition to the obvious tuition cost, can include many fees, room and board, daily meals at clinical sites, books, uniforms, and malpractice insurance. Students will also have to purchase nursing supplies, such as stethoscopes, bandage scissors, and thermometers. Students must also consider the cost of vehicle maintenance, personal health costs, and the costs of life outside of nursing school.

Financial Assistance Considerations

The first step for students pursuing financial aid is to consult with their nursing program's financial aid department. Before accepting financial aid, students must be sure to understand fully all of the terms of the loan. Financial aid may require students to maintain a certain grade-point average or number of credit hours. While student loans are usually associated with lower interest rates, they must be repaid upon graduation from the nursing program (earlier if the student fails or withdraws from the nursing program). Students who do not repay the loan can be impacted by a negative credit score and, in more severe cases, forfeiture of their license to practice nursing. In some cases, students may be eligible to receive grants or scholarships that do not require repayment.

Sociology

Sociology is the study of humans as they coexist in groups. One of the basic principles of sociology is that humans will behave in the same manner as those around them. Sociologists study the development of society and social behavior among humans, origins, organizations, and institutions. They may study one group or institution as a self-contained entity or as part of a greater whole. Sociology also concerns itself with the question of whether nature or nurture exerts greater influence on the existence of a human. It may be said that a sociologist studies the various processes that create and maintain a system of social structure.

Psychology

Psychology is the study of the mental processes and behavior of an individual. Psychologists may study the general characteristics of individuals or large groups. The field of psychology can be divided into applied and experimental areas. Certain psychologists examine mental processes. Other psychologists examine the elements of consciousness, such as mental activity, free will, and memory. The field of social psychology combines psychology and sociology. It is the study of the interactions that occur between individuals and groups. It also is the study of the effects of groups on the behaviors and attitudes of the individual.

Ethics

Ethical principles should be understood and used by nurses. When applied correctly, ethical principles can facilitate decision making in all facets of life. Nursing especially is a profession in which ethics play a large role. The patients trust that the nurses will always make decisions that are in the best interest of the patient. The study of science and medicine can equip an individual with the skills necessary to save or improve a person's life; however, ethics give the individual the ability to make decisions regarding matters of life and death. Nurses must always be aware of the impact their behavior and actions will have on their patients.

Ethical Principle of Beneficence

Beneficence is the practice of always helping other people. The definition of the word *beneficent* is *doing or producing good, especially through the acts of charity and kindness.* This principle is central to the role of health care providers that it is part of the Hippocratic Oath sworn by medical doctors. In the field of ethics, the term *beneficence* has an additional component that requires that no intentional harm be done to another person. In other words, nonmaleficence is an essential component of beneficence. There are three theories regarding beneficence: Humes' theory, utilitarian theory, and Kant's theory. Hume's theory is that the motive behind an act of kindness determines the validity of the act. Utilitarian theory states that beneficence is simply the drive to create happiness through kindness or unhappiness through unkindness. Kant's theory states that beneficence is motivated by a sense of duty.

Ethical Principle of Justice

The ethical principle of justice centers on the fair and equal treatment of all individuals. Nurses must constantly evaluate their own motives when treating patients. Each patient should receive the same degree of attention, compassion, and care. Nurses must remember to speak confidentially about patients, as well as to maintain discretion about a patient's condition. In the health care field, questions of ethical justice often arise because of insurance and patient needs. Oftentimes, a patient will need a specific type of care but does not have the financial resources to pay for it. There is also the question of compensatory justice, in which one individual or group of individuals has been harmed by the actions of another.

Ethical Principle of Autonomy

In the most basic sense, the ethical principle of autonomy refers to a patient's right to choose a course of action and follow or change it as they see fit. In order for patients to choose freely, they must be provided with the appropriate information. Medical facilities often attempt to uphold the ethical principle of autonomy by providing patients with informed consent documents. Autonomy requires that patients be allowed to decide and act without pressure or coercion from another party. Medical professionals can aid in the freedom to choose by making sure that patients have adequate information about the choices available to them. Medical professionals can aid in the freedom to act by ensuring that the patient and the patient's family understand the importance of respecting the autonomy of the individual.

Mass Casualties
It seems that the increasing technological capabilities of the modern world are accompanied by the increasing threat of mass devastation. Entire cities can be built of towers that reach hundreds of stories in height. With all of this development comes an increase in the risk of mass injury. Imagine that you are a triage nurse working the emergency room when over 300 seriously injured patients are routed to your hospital. How do you decide who is treated first? Nurses must use the utilitarian principle of ethics, in which the greatest good must be done for the greatest number of people.

Bioethical Issues
The most intense bioethical issues faced by nurses involve the beginning and end of life. Modern technology has introduced in vitro fertilization, contraception, abortion, genetic modification, cloning, and surrogate mothers. All of these are useful tools, but each comes with its own set of ethical dilemmas. This is also the case with issues surrounding the end of life. Ethical concerns include euthanasia, the definition of death, death through outside intervention, and the handling of patients with diseases brought about by avoidable behaviors. For example, imagine that a hospital with a limited staff has two patients suffering from lung cancer. They are the same age with similar backgrounds. Now imagine one patient is a lifelong smoker, while the other has never smoked. If the hospital only has resources to treat one of those patients, which one should they choose?

Testing

Critical Thinking Skills

Critical thinking is a skill that nurses must use on a regular basis. Critical thinking is a combination of scientific knowledge and the logical application of that knowledge. In the course of daily life, people are constantly faced with opportunities to use critical thinking skills. An individual may be presented with a problem for which they must find the best possible solution. In order to do so, the individual must consider a variety of possible solutions. They must understand the consequences associated with each solution and the manner in which the solution will resolve the problem. Students should carefully read and analyze each possible response for each test question. By understanding fully all of the options available, students can select the best solution.

Standardized Testing Tips

In addition to critical thinking, a variety of testing strategies can be utilized in standardized testing. For example, in a timed multiple-choice test, students should answer the questions of which they are certain, skipping over questions that require more time to think. This will allow the student to devote the appropriate amount of time to harder questions, without running the risk of earning a lower score for running out of time. Test-takers should read questions carefully, looking out for words such as *first* or *usually*. These words can be very important when selecting the best response. When faced with a tough question, students should avoid selecting answers that use the terms *always* and *never*. Correct answers are most often worded with less absolute language, such as the phrases *in most cases* or *usually*. Students should also be cautious when answering questions that imply a cause-and-effect relationship. When selecting an answer for this type of question, avoid options that state one thing is causing another. Instead, select a more conservative option that states the two things are somehow connected.

Process of Elimination

Standardized tests are most commonly organized into questions with four possible answer choices. For each question, there is a 1 in 4 chance (25%) that the student will select the correct answer. This also means there is a 3 in 4 chance (75%) that the student will select the wrong answer. The odds seem to favor the student answering incorrectly. By simply eliminating the obviously incorrect answers, students can increase the odds of selecting the correct answer. If there are four possible answer choices, eliminating two of those answers will give the student a 50% chance of answering the question correctly. By the simple process of elimination, a student can increase his chances of answering a question correctly even if he knows very little about the subject.

Multiple-Choice Questions

In standardized multiple-choice tests, there are three levels of test questions: recall, application, and analysis.

Recall Questions

In standardized multiple-choice tests, there are three levels of test questions: recall, application, and analysis. Recall questions require the test-taker simply to remember a piece of information. An example of a recall question is a definition. The question may ask the student to select the best definition of a word that is either contained within a sentence or provided in a more straightforward form. Recall questions will not require the student to analyze or apply knowledge. Once a student identifies a recall question, she can answer it directly (if she knows the correct answer) or she can begin to eliminate incorrect answers to increase her odds of answering correctly.

Memory Aids

When answering a recall-level question, students often either know the answer or do not. When a student does not immediately know the correct answer, he can try a memory trick. Namely, he should move on to another question or think of something else entirely. By giving his mind a distraction, and then returning to the troublesome question, the answer will often become clear. Students may also use visual association when learning material. For example, in order to remember that arteries carry blood away from the heart, a student might picture the heart as a museum filled with art, which is stolen by a thief. By picturing a thief stealing art, the student associates the word *art* with the word *arteries*, thus remembering that arteries carry blood away from the heart. Another method is the comparison strategy. By finding similarities between pieces of information, students can more readily retain knowledge. For example, arteries carry blood away from the heart. Both *artery* and *away* begin with the letter *a*.

Application Questions
Application questions require that students use the knowledge they have learned. Students may be asked to apply the knowledge they have acquired from textbooks and apply it to a real-life situation. For example, a question may provide a brief scenario described in paragraph form. A question will ask the student to use the information presented in the paragraph. In general, the questions will be asked in the form of "if you know this about X, what can be assumed about Y?" These questions will present all of the information students need within the question. By carefully reading the questions and examining the answer choices, students should be able to locate the correct answer.

Analysis Questions
Analysis-level questions are the most complex of the three levels. For this type of problem, students must carefully read the question, dissect it, and then study the interaction between its various parts. Students may find that analysis-level questions require them to identify what piece of information is missing. Students should read each answer choice provided and examine how well that piece fits into the puzzle. The student should consider whether the answer choice actually provides a solution, or whether it simply produces more questions. As with all test questions, students improve their chances of success by eliminating the obviously incorrect choices.

Preparing for Standardized Exams
Standardized testing can be a stressful situation for students. It is crucial that students begin studying material early so that they have plenty of time to prepare. By studying early, students can avoid all-night cram sessions that deprive them of sleep, nutrition, and mental health. Students should avoid overly emotional interactions prior to a test, because this can cause increased anxiety, which could lead to decreased performance. At least ten days prior to the test, the student should begin taking multi-vitamins, eating properly, getting plenty of rest, and exercising. All of these things will give the body what it needs to perform at its highest level on test day.

Personality Profile

The Admission Assessment test will include 15 items designed to gauge your personality type. Although there are no wrong answers to these questions, it is a good idea to learn the conceptual framework underlying the personality profile. The primary distinction made by these questions is between the extroverted and introverted personality types.

Extroverted Personality Type
The extroverted personality type is characterized by a desire to be around other people. Extroverted individuals draw energy from their interaction with others. Extroverts are likely to enjoy social gatherings, and are most successful when working in collaboration with other people. Extroverts are more talkative, gregarious, and assertive of their own desires than are introverts.

Introverted PersonalityType
The introverted personality type is characterized by a desire to be alone and away from other people. Introversion should not be confused with antisocial personality disorder; there is no pathology associated with normal introversion. Introverts tend to be imaginative and thoughtful, and often enjoy activities like reading, distance running, and writing. Introverts tend to be more successful when they are allowed to work independently. For introverts, social interaction can be depleting and exhausting. Introverts often report a need to "recharge" by spending time alone. Introverts prefer to observe activities before participating, and tend to be more analytical than extroverts.

Learning styles

The Admission Assessment will include 14 items designed to gauge your learning style. As with the personality profile, there are no incorrect answers to these questions. However, it is a good idea to be acquainted with the seven common learning styles: spatial, auditory-musical, linguistic, kinesthetic, mathematical, interpersonal, and intrapersonal.

Spatial Learning Style
Students with the spatial learning style (also known as the visual learning style) learn best by using pictures and images. They find it is easier to retain information that is presented in a table or chart. They prefer to use a map to orient themselves rather than to rely on a set of written directions. Color coding information is a helpful method of teaching for student with this learning style.

Auditory-Musical Learning Style
Students with the auditory-musical learning style (also known as the aural learning style) learn best by using sound, and especially music. These students have a natural sense of rhythm and harmony, and find it easy to remember the words to songs. Often, these students unconsciously drum out a beat on their desk or keep up a constant rhythm of toe taps under their chair. They can improve their retention of new information by placing it into a rhyme or setting it to a familiar tune. These students often have success using mnemonics based on popular songs.

Linguistic Learning Style
Students with the linguistic learning style (also known as the verbal learning style) learn best by using words, whether spoken or written. These students like to express themselves with words, and are very receptive to the language used in texts and by teachers. They will also have a natural facility for wordplay, and will enjoy word-based puzzles and games. Students with a linguistic learning style will find it easy to retain the information they read, and should be able to express themselves clearly in writing. They enjoy reading texts aloud, and benefit from mnemonics based on wordplay and common expressions.

Kinesthetic Learning Style
Students with the kinesthetic learning style (also known as the physical learning style) learn best by using physical movement and gesture. These students retain information that they receive through their sense of touch. Often, students with a kinesthetic style of learning will be able to retain spoken information better when their hands are kept occupied. For instance, studies have shown that kinesthetic learners pick up their multiplication tables faster when they are allowed to bounce a ball while practicing. These students also love to make models and three-dimensional representations of the things they have learned.

Mathematical Learning Style
Students with the mathematical learning style (also known as the logical learning style) learn best by using systems of logic and analytical reasoning. These students are great at recognizing patterns, and are quick to discern the logical system underlying a set of information. These students prefer to work through problems in a systematic manner, and thrive in highly structured learning environments. A student with a mathematical learning style will appreciate being given a list of the tasks to be accomplished over a certain interval. These students excel in the sciences and any other area that calls for rigorous, systematic thinking.

Interpersonal Learning Style
Students with the interpersonal learning style (also known as the social learning style) learn best when working in collaboration with other people. These students are good communicators, and have no problem making their meaning plain to other people. They are also sensitive to the concerns of other people, and have a genuine interest in preserving harmony within the work group. Interpersonal learners work best in groups, and often exhibit strong leadership skills. These students enjoy role-playing exercises and peer-review assignments. They may become frustrated or bored when asked to work alone for a long time.

Intrapersonal Learning Style

Students with the intrapersonal learning style (also known as the solitary learning style) learn best by themselves. These students become frustrated when working in a group, and prefer to act independently. They often need a period of reflection before initiating an activity. They often excel at reading and writing. Student with an intrapersonal learning style will thrive in structured learning environments, and will prefer consistency to chaos. These students may become over-stimulated by contact with other people, and require frequent opportunities to recharge with solitude and contemplation. Intrapersonal learners tend to be reserved and thoughtful, but capable of developing strong relationships with a few select peers.

Practice Test

Reading Comprehension Questions

Questions 1 to 4 pertain to the following passage:

It is most likely that you have never had diphtheria. You probably don't even know anyone who has suffered from this disease. In fact, you may not even know what diphtheria is. Similarly, diseases like whooping cough, measles, mumps, and rubella may all be unfamiliar to you. In the nineteenth and early twentieth centuries, these illnesses struck hundreds of thousands of people in the United States each year, mostly children, and tens of thousands of people died. The names of these diseases were frightening household words. Today, they are all but forgotten. That change happened largely because of vaccines.

You probably have been vaccinated against diphtheria. You may even have been exposed to the bacterium that causes it, but the vaccine prepared your body to fight off the disease so quickly that you were unaware of the infection. Vaccines take advantage of your body's natural ability to learn how to combat many disease-causing germs, or microbes. What's more, your body remembers how to protect itself from the microbes it has encountered before. Collectively, the parts of your body that remember and repel microbes are called the immune system. Without the proper functioning of the immune system, the simplest illness—even the common cold—could quickly turn deadly.

On average, your immune system needs more than a week to learn how to fight off an unfamiliar microbe. Sometimes, that isn't enough time. Strong microbes can spread through your body faster than the immune system can fend them off. Your body often gains the upper hand after a few weeks, but in the meantime you are sick. Certain microbes are so virulent that they can overwhelm or escape your natural defenses. In those situations, vaccines can make all the difference.

Traditional vaccines contain either parts of microbes or whole microbes that have been altered so that they don't cause disease. When your immune system confronts these harmless versions of the germs, it quickly clears them from your body. In other words, vaccines trick your immune system in order to teach your body important lessons about how to defeat its opponents.

1. What is the main idea of the passage?
    a. The nineteenth and early twentieth centuries were a dark period for medicine.
    b. You have probably never had diphtheria.
    c. Traditional vaccines contain altered microbes.
    d. Vaccines help the immune system function properly.

2. Which statement is *not* a detail from the passage?
    a. Vaccines contain microbe parts or altered microbes.
    b. The immune system typically needs a week to learn how to fight a new disease.
    c. The symptoms of disease do not emerge until the body has learned how to fight the microbe.
    d. A hundred years ago, children were at the greatest risk of dying from now-treatable diseases.

3. What is the meaning of the word *virulent* as it is used in the third paragraph?
    a. tiny
    b. malicious
    c. contagious
    d. annoying

4. What is the author's primary purpose in writing the essay?
   a. to entertain
   b. to persuade
   c. to inform
   d. to analyze

Questions 5 to 8 pertain to the following passage :
   Foodborne illnesses are contracted by eating food or drinking beverages contaminated with bacteria, parasites, or viruses. Harmful chemicals can also cause foodborne illnesses if they have contaminated food during harvesting or processing. Foodborne illnesses can cause symptoms ranging from upset stomach to diarrhea, fever, vomiting, abdominal cramps, and dehydration. Most foodborne infections are undiagnosed and unreported, though the Centers for Disease Control and Prevention estimates that every year about 76 million people in the United States become ill from pathogens in food. About 5,000 of these people die.
   Harmful bacteria are the most common cause of foodborne illness. Some bacteria may be present at the point of purchase. Raw foods are the most common source of foodborne illnesses because they are not sterile; examples include raw meat and poultry contaminated during slaughter. Seafood may become contaminated during harvest or processing. One in 10,000 eggs may be contaminated with Salmonella inside the shell. Produce, such as spinach, lettuce, tomatoes, sprouts, and melons, can become contaminated with Salmonella, Shigella, or Escherichia coli (E. coli). Contamination can occur during growing, harvesting, processing, storing, shipping, or final preparation. Sources of produce contamination vary, as these foods are grown in soil and can become contaminated during growth, processing, or distribution. Contamination may also occur during food preparation in a restaurant or a home kitchen. The most common form of contamination from handled foods is the calicivirus, also called the Norwalk-like virus.
   When food is cooked and left out for more than two hours at room temperature, bacteria can multiply quickly. Most bacteria don't produce an odor or change in color or texture, so they can be impossible to detect. Freezing food slows or stops bacteria's growth, but does not destroy the bacteria. The microbes can become reactivated when the food is thawed. Refrigeration also can slow the growth of some bacteria. Thorough cooking is required to destroy the bacteria.

5. What is the subject of the passage?
   a. foodborne illnesses
   b. the dangers of uncooked food
   c. bacteria
   d. proper food preparation

6. Which statement is *not* a detail from the passage?
   a. Every year, more than 70 million Americans contract some form of foodborne illness.
   b. Once food is cooked, it cannot cause illness.
   c. Refrigeration can slow the growth of some bacteria.
   d. The most common form of contamination in handled foods is calicivirus.

7. What is the meaning of the word *pathogens* as it is used in the first paragraph?
   a. diseases
   b. vaccines
   c. disease-causing substances
   d. foods

8. What is the meaning of the word *sterile* as it is used in the second paragraph?
    a. free of bacteria
    b. healthy
    c. delicious
    d. impotent

Questions 9 to 12 pertain to the following passage:

There are a number of health problems related to bleeding in the esophagus and stomach. Stomach acid can cause inflammation and bleeding at the lower end of the esophagus. This condition, usually associated with the symptom of heartburn, is called esophagitis, or inflammation of the esophagus. Sometimes a muscle between the esophagus and stomach fails to close properly and allows the return of food and stomach juices into the esophagus, which can lead to esophagitis. In another unrelated condition, enlarged veins (varices) at the lower end of the esophagus rupture and bleed massively. Cirrhosis of the liver is the most common cause of esophageal varices. Esophageal bleeding can be caused by a tear in the lining of the esophagus (Mallory-Weiss syndrome). Mallory-Weiss syndrome usually results from vomiting, but may also be caused by increased pressure in the abdomen from coughing, hiatal hernia, or childbirth. Esophageal cancer can cause bleeding.

The stomach is a frequent site of bleeding. Infections with Helicobacter pylori (H. pylori), alcohol, aspirin, aspirin-containing medicines, and various other medicines (such as nonsteroidal anti-inflammatory drugs [NSAIDs]—particularly those used for arthritis) can cause stomach ulcers or inflammation (gastritis). The stomach is often the site of ulcer disease. Acute or chronic ulcers may enlarge and erode through a blood vessel, causing bleeding. Also, patients suffering from burns, shock, head injuries, cancer, or those who have undergone extensive surgery may develop stress ulcers. Bleeding can also occur from benign tumors or cancer of the stomach, although these disorders usually do not cause massive bleeding.

9. What is the main idea of the passage?
    a. The digestive system is complex.
    b. Of all the digestive organs, the stomach is the most prone to bleeding.
    c. Both the esophagus and the stomach are subject to bleeding problems.
    d. Esophagitis afflicts the young and old alike.

10. Which statement is *not* a detail from the passage?
    a. Alcohol can cause stomach bleeding.
    b. Ulcer disease rarely occurs in the stomach.
    c. Benign tumors rarely result in massive bleeding.
    d. Childbirth is one cause of Mallory-Weiss syndrome.

11. What is the meaning of the word *rupture* as it is used in the first paragraph?
    a. tear
    b. collapse
    c. implode
    d. detach

12. What is the meaning of the word *erode* as it is used in the second paragraph?
    a. avoid
    b. divorce
    c. contain
    d. wear away

Questions 13 to 16 pertain to the following passage:

We met Kathy Blake while she was taking a stroll in the park . . . by herself. What's so striking about this is that Kathy is completely blind, and she has been for more than 30 years.

The diagnosis from her doctor was retinitis pigmentosa, or RP. It's an incurable genetic disease that leads to progressive visual loss. Photoreceptive cells in the retina slowly start to die, leaving the patient visually impaired.

"Life was great the year before I was diagnosed," Kathy said. "I had just started a new job; I just bought my first new car. I had just started dating my now-husband. Life was good. The doctor had told me that there was some good news and some bad news. 'The bad news is you are going to lose your vision; the good news is we don't think you are going to go totally blind.' Unfortunately, I did lose all my vision within about 15 years."

Two years ago, Kathy got a glimmer of hope. She heard about an artificial retina being developed in Los Angeles. It was experimental, but Kathy was the perfect candidate.

Dr. Mark Humayun is a retinal surgeon and biomedical engineer. "A good candidate for the artificial retina device is a person who is blind because of retinal blindness," he said. "They've lost the rods and cones, the light-sensing cells of the eye, but the rest of the circuitry is relatively intact. In the simplest rendition, this device basically takes a blind person and hooks them up to a camera."

It may sound like the stuff of science fiction . . . and just a few years ago it was. A camera is built into a pair of glasses, sending radio signals to a tiny chip in the back of the retina. The chip, small enough to fit on a fingertip, is implanted surgically and stimulates the nerves that lead to the vision center of the brain. Kathy is one of twenty patients who have undergone surgery and use the device.

It has been about two years since the surgery, and Kathy still comes in for weekly testing at the University of Southern California's medical campus. She scans back and forth with specially made, camera-equipped glasses until she senses objects on a screen and then touches the objects. The low-resolution image from the camera is still enough to make out the black stripes on the screen. Impulses are sent from the camera to the 60 receptors that are on the chip in her retina. So, what is Kathy seeing?

"I see flashes of light that indicate a contrast from light to dark—very similar to a camera flash, probably not quite as bright because it's not hurting my eye at all," she replied.

Humayun underscored what a breakthrough this is and how a patient adjusts. "If you've been blind for 30 or 50 years, (and) all of a sudden you get this device, there is a period of learning," he said. "Your brain needs to learn. And it's literally like seeing a baby crawl—to a child walk—to an adult run."

While hardly perfect, the device works best in bright light or where there is a lot of contrast. Kathy takes the device home. The software that runs the device can be upgraded. So, as the software is upgraded, her vision improves. Recently, she was outside with her husband on a moonlit night and saw something she hadn't seen for a long time.

"I scanned up in the sky (and) I got a big flash, right where the moon was, and pointed it out. I can't even remember how many years ago it's been that I would have ever been able to do that."

This technology has a bright future. The current chip has a resolution of 60 pixels. Humayun says that number could be increased to more than a thousand in the next version.

"I think it will be extremely exciting if they can recognize their loved ones' faces and be able to see what their wife or husband or their grandchildren look like, which they haven't seen," said Humayun.

Kathy dreams of a day when blindness like hers will be a distant memory. "My eye disease is hereditary," she said. "My three daughters happen to be fine, but I want to know that if my grandchildren ever have a problem, they will have something to give them some vision."

13. What is the primary subject of the passage?
   a. a new artificial retina
   b. Kathy Blake
   c. hereditary disease
   d. Dr. Mark Humayun

14. What is the meaning of the word *progressive* as it is used in the second paragraph?
   a. selective
   b. gradually increasing
   c. diminishing
   d. disabling

15. Which statement is *not* a detail from the passage?
   a. The use of an artificial retina requires a special pair of glasses.
   b. Retinal blindness is the inability to perceive light.
   c. Retinitis pigmentosa is curable.
   d. The artificial retina performs best in bright light.

16. What is the author's intention in writing the essay?
   a. to persuade
   b. to entertain
   c. to analyze
   d. to inform

Questions 17 to 21 pertain to the following passage:

Usher syndrome is the most common condition that affects both hearing and vision. The major symptoms of Usher syndrome are hearing loss and an eye disorder called retinitis pigmentosa, or RP. Retinitis pigmentosa causes night blindness and a loss of peripheral vision (side vision) through the progressive degeneration of the retina. The retina, which is crucial for vision, is a light-sensitive tissue at the back of the eye. As RP progresses, the field of vision narrows, until only central vision (the ability to see straight ahead) remains. Many people with Usher syndrome also have severe balance problems.

There are three clinical types of Usher syndrome. In the United States, types 1 and 2 are the most common. Together, they account for approximately 90 to 95 percent of all cases of juvenile Usher syndrome. Approximately three to six percent of all deaf and hearing-disabled children have Usher syndrome. In developed countries, such as the United States, about four in every 100,000 newborns have Usher syndrome.

Usher syndrome is inherited as an autosomal recessive trait. The term autosomal means that the mutated gene is not located on either of the chromosomes that determine sex; in other words, both males and females can have the disorder and can pass it along to a child. The word recessive means that in order to have Usher syndrome, an individual must receive a mutated form of the Usher syndrome gene from each parent. If a child has a mutation in one Usher syndrome gene but the other gene is normal, he or she should have normal vision and hearing. Individuals with a mutation in a gene that can cause an autosomal recessive disorder are called carriers, because they carry the mutated gene but show no symptoms of the disorder. If both parents are carriers of a mutated gene for Usher syndrome, they will have a one-in-four chance of producing a child with Usher syndrome.

Usually, parents who have normal hearing and vision do not know if they are carriers of an Usher syndrome gene mutation. Currently, it is not possible to determine whether an individual without a family history of Usher syndrome is a carrier. Scientists at the National Institute on Deafness and

Other Communication Disorders (NIDCD) are hoping to change this, however, as they learn more about the genes responsible for Usher syndrome.

17. What is the main idea of the passage?
    a. Usher syndrome is an inherited condition that affects hearing and vision.
    b. Some people are carriers of Usher syndrome.
    c. Usher syndrome typically skips a generation.
    d. Scientists hope to develop a test for detecting the carriers of Usher syndrome.

18. What is the meaning of the word *symptoms* as it is used in the first paragraph?
    a. qualifications
    b. conditions
    c. disorders
    d. perceptible signs

19. Which statement is *not* a detail from the passage?
    a. Types 1 and 2 Usher syndrome are the most common in the United States.
    b. Usher syndrome affects both hearing and smell.
    c. Right now, there is no way to identify a carrier of Usher syndrome.
    d. Central vision is the ability to see straight ahead.

20. What is the meaning of the word *juvenile* as it is used in the second paragraph?
    a. bratty
    b. serious
    c. occurring in children
    d. improper

21. What is the meaning of the word *mutated* as it is used in the third paragraph?
    a. selected
    b. altered
    c. composed
    d. destroyed

Questions 22 to 27 pertain to the following passage:
The immune system is a network of cells, tissues, and organs that defends the body against attacks by foreign invaders. These invaders are primarily microbes—tiny organisms such as bacteria, parasites, and fungi—that can cause infections. Viruses also cause infections, but are too primitive to be classified as living organisms. The human body provides an ideal environment for many microbes. It is the immune system's job to keep the microbes out or destroy them.
The immune system is amazingly complex. It can recognize and remember millions of different enemies, and it can secrete fluids and cells to wipe out nearly all of them. The secret to its success is an elaborate and dynamic communications network. Millions of cells, organized into sets and subsets, gather and transfer information in response to an infection. Once immune cells receive the alarm, they produce powerful chemicals that help to regulate their own growth and behavior, enlist other immune cells, and direct the new recruits to trouble spots.
Although scientists have learned much about the immune system, they continue to puzzle over how the body destroys invading microbes, infected cells, and tumors without harming healthy tissues. New technologies for identifying individual immune cells are now allowing scientists to determine quickly which targets are triggering an immune response. Improvements in microscopy are permitting the first-ever observations of living B cells, T cells, and other cells as they interact within lymph nodes and other body tissues.

In addition, scientists are rapidly unraveling the genetic blueprints that direct the human immune response, as well as those that dictate the biology of bacteria, viruses, and parasites. The combination of new technology with expanded genetic information will no doubt reveal even more about how the body protects itself from disease.

22. What is the main idea of the passage?
    a. Scientists fully understand the immune system.
    b. The immune system triggers the production of fluids.
    c. The body is under constant invasion by malicious microbes.
    d. The immune system protects the body from infection.

23. Which statement is *not* a detail from the passage?
    a. Most invaders of the body are microbes.
    b. The immune system relies on excellent communication.
    c. Viruses are extremely sophisticated.
    d. The cells of the immune system are organized.

24. What is the meaning of the word *ideal* as it is used in the first paragraph?
    a. thoughtful
    b. confined
    c. hostile
    d. perfect

25. Which statement is *not* a detail from the passage?
    a. Scientists can now see T cells.
    b. The immune system ignores tumors.
    c. The ability of the immune system to fight disease without harming the body remains mysterious.
    d. The immune system remembers millions of different invaders.

26. What is the meaning of the word *enlist* as it is used in the second paragraph?
    a. call into service
    b. write down
    c. send away
    d. put across

27. What is the author's primary purpose in writing the essay?
    a. to persuade
    b. to analyze
    c. to inform
    d. to entertain

Questions 28 to 31 pertain to the following passage:

The federal government regulates dietary supplements through the United States Food and Drug Administration (FDA). The regulations for dietary supplements are not the same as those for prescription or over-the-counter drugs. In general, the regulations for dietary supplements are less strict.

To begin with, a manufacturer does not have to prove the safety and effectiveness of a dietary supplement before it is marketed. A manufacturer is permitted to say that a dietary supplement addresses a nutrient deficiency, supports health, or is linked to a particular body function (such as immunity), if there is research to support the claim. Such a claim must be followed by the words

"This statement has not been evaluated by the Food and Drug Administration. This product is not intended to diagnose, treat, cure, or prevent any disease."

Also, manufacturers are expected to follow certain good manufacturing practices (GMPs) to ensure that dietary supplements are processed consistently and meet quality standards. Requirements for GMPs went into effect in 2008 for large manufacturers and are being phased in for small manufacturers through 2010.

Once a dietary supplement is on the market, the FDA monitors safety and product information, such as label claims and package inserts. If it finds a product to be unsafe, it can take action against the manufacturer and/or distributor and may issue a warning or require that the product be removed from the marketplace. The Federal Trade Commission (FTC) is responsible for regulating product advertising; it requires that all information be truthful and not misleading. The federal government has taken legal action against a number of dietary supplement promoters or Web sites that promote or sell dietary supplements because they have made false or deceptive statements about their products or because marketed products have proven to be unsafe.

28. What is the main idea of the passage?
   a. Manufacturers of dietary supplements have to follow good manufacturing practices.
   b. The FDA has a special program for regulating dietary supplements.
   c. The federal government prosecutes those who mislead the general public.
   d. The FDA is part of the federal government.

29. Which statement is *not* a detail from the passage?
   a. Promoters of dietary supplements can make any claims that are supported by research.
   b. GMP requirements for large manufacturers went into effect in 2008.
   c. Product advertising is regulated by the FTC.
   d. The FDA does not monitor products after they enter the market.

30. What is the meaning of the phrase *phased in* as it is used in the third paragraph?
   a. stunned into silence
   b. confused
   c. implemented in stages
   d. legalized

31. What is the meaning of the word *deceptive* as it is used in the fifth paragraph?
   a. misleading
   b. malicious
   c. illegal
   d. irritating

Questions 32 to 35 pertain to the following passage:

Anemia is a condition in which there is an abnormally low number of red blood cells (RBCs). This condition also can occur if the RBCs don't contain enough hemoglobin, the iron-rich protein that makes the blood red. Hemoglobin helps RBCs carry oxygen from the lungs to the rest of the body. Anemia can be accompanied by low numbers of RBCs, white blood cells (WBCs), and platelets. Red blood cells are disc-shaped and look like doughnuts without holes in the center. They carry oxygen and remove carbon dioxide (a waste product) from your body. These cells are made in the bone marrow and live for about 120 days in the bloodstream. Platelets and WBCs also are made in the bone marrow. White blood cells help fight infection. Platelets stick together to seal small cuts or breaks on the blood vessel walls and to stop bleeding.

If you are anemic, your body doesn't get enough oxygenated blood. As a result, you may feel tired or have other symptoms. Severe or long-lasting anemia can damage the heart, brain, and other organs of the body. Very severe anemia may even cause death.

Anemia has three main causes: blood loss, lack of RBC production, or high rates of RBC destruction. Many types of anemia are mild, brief, and easily treated. Some types can be prevented with a healthy diet or treated with dietary supplements. However, certain types of anemia may be severe, long lasting, and life threatening if not diagnosed and treated.

If you have the signs or symptoms of anemia, you should see your doctor to find out whether you have the condition. Treatment will depend on the cause and severity of the anemia.

32. What is the main idea of the passage?
   a. Anemia presents in a number of forms.
   b. Anemia is a potentially dangerous condition characterized by low numbers of RBCs.
   c. Anemia is a deficiency of WBCs and platelets.
   d. Anemia is a treatable condition.

33. Which statement is *not* a detail from the passage?
   a. There are different methods for treating anemia.
   b. Red blood cells remove carbon dioxide from the body.
   c. Platelets are made in the bone marrow.
   d. Anemia is rarely caused by blood loss.

34. What is the meaning of the word *oxygenated* as it is used in the third paragraph?
   a. containing low amounts of oxygen
   b. containing no oxygen
   c. consisting entirely of oxygen
   d. containing high amounts of oxygen

35. What is the meaning of the word *severity* as it is used in the fifth paragraph?
   a. seriousness
   b. disconnectedness
   c. truth
   d. swiftness

Questions 36 to 39 pertain to the following passage :

Contrary to previous reports, drinking four or more cups of coffee a day does not put women at risk of rheumatoid arthritis (RA), according to a new study partially funded by the National Institute of Arthritis and Musculoskeletal and Skin Diseases (NIAMS). The study concluded that there is little evidence to support a connection between consuming coffee or tea and the risk of RA among women.

Rheumatoid arthritis is an inflammatory autoimmune disease that affects the joints. It results in pain, stiffness, swelling, joint damage, and loss of function. Inflammation most often affects the hands and feet and tends to be symmetrical. About one percent of the U.S. population has rheumatoid arthritis.

Elizabeth W. Karlson, M.D., and her colleagues at Harvard Medical School and Brigham and Women's Hospital in Boston, Massachusetts, used the Nurses' Health Study, a long-term investigation of nurses' diseases, lifestyles, and health practices, to examine possible links between caffeinated beverages and RA risk. The researchers were able to follow up more than 90 percent of the original pool of 83,124 participants who answered a 1980 food frequency questionnaire, and no links were found. They also considered changes in diet and habits over a prolonged period of time, and when the results were adjusted for other factors, such as cigarette

- 99 -

smoking, alcohol consumption, and oral contraceptive use, the outcome still showed no relationship between caffeine consumption and risk of RA.

Previous research had suggested an association between consuming coffee or tea and RA risk. According to Dr. Karlson, the data supporting that conclusion were inconsistent. Because the information in the older studies was collected at only one time, she says, consideration was not given to the other factors associated with RA, such as cigarette smoking and changes in diet and lifestyle over a follow-up period. The new study presents a more accurate picture of caffeine and RA risk.

36. What is the main idea of the passage?
   a. In the past, doctors have cautioned older women to avoid caffeinated beverages.
   b. Rheumatoid arthritis affects the joints of older women.
   c. A recent study found no link between caffeine consumption and RA among women.
   d. Cigarette smoking increases the incidence of RA.

37. Which statement is *not* a detail from the passage?
   a. Alcohol consumption is linked with RA.
   b. The original data for the study came from a 1980 questionnaire.
   c. Rheumatoid arthritis most often affects the hands and feet.
   d. This study included tens of thousands of participants.

38. What is the meaning of the word *symmetrical* as it is used in the second paragraph?
   a. affecting both sides of the body in corresponding fashion
   b. impossible to treat
   c. sensitive to the touch
   d. asymptomatic

39. What is the author's primary purpose in writing the essay?
   a. to entertain
   b. to inform
   c. to analyze
   d. to persuade

Questions 40 to 43 refer to the following passage:

Exercise is vital at every age for healthy bones. Not only does exercise improve bone health, but it also increases muscle strength, coordination, and balance, and it leads to better overall health. Exercise is especially important for preventing and treating osteoporosis.

Like muscle, bone is living tissue that responds to exercise by becoming stronger. Young women and men who exercise regularly generally achieve greater peak bone mass (maximum bone density and strength) than those who do not. For most people, bone mass peaks during the third decade of life. After that time, we can begin to lose bone. Women and men older than age 20 can help prevent bone loss with regular exercise. Exercise maintains muscle strength, coordination, and balance, which in turn prevent falls and related fractures. This is especially important for older adults and people with osteoporosis.

Weight-bearing exercise is the best kind of exercise for bones, which forces the muscle to work against gravity. Some examples of weight-bearing exercises are weight training, walking, hiking, jogging, climbing stairs, tennis, and dancing. Swimming and bicycling, on the other hand, are not weight-bearing exercises. Although these activities help build and maintain strong muscles and have excellent cardiovascular benefits, they are not the best exercise for bones.

40. What is the main idea of the passage?
    a. Weight-bearing exercise is the best for bones.
    b. Exercise increases balance.
    c. Exercise improves bone health.
    d. Women benefit from regular exercise more than men.

41. What is the meaning of the word *vital* as it is used in the first paragraph?
    a. deadly
    b. important
    c. rejected
    d. nourishing

42. Which statement is *not* a detail from the passage?
    a. Tennis is a form of weight-bearing exercise.
    b. Most people reach peak bone mass in their twenties.
    c. Swimming is not good for the bones.
    d. Bone is a living tissue.

43. What is the meaning of the word *fractures* as it is used in the second paragraph?
    a. breaks
    b. agreements
    c. tiffs
    d. fevers

Questions 44 to 47 pertain to the following passage :
Searching for medical information can be confusing, especially for first-timers. However, if you are patient and stick to it, you can find a wealth of information. Your community library is a good place to start your search for medical information. Before going to the library, you may find it helpful to make a list of topics you want information about and questions you have. Your list of topics and questions will make it easier for the librarian to direct you to the best resources.
Many community libraries have a collection of basic medical references. These references may include medical dictionaries or encyclopedias, drug information handbooks, basic medical and nursing textbooks, and directories of physicians and medical specialists (listings of doctors). You may also find magazine articles on a certain topic. Look in the Reader's Guide to Periodical Literature for articles on health and medicine from consumer magazines.
Infotrac, a CD-ROM computer database available at libraries or on the Web, indexes hundreds of popular magazines and newspapers, as well as medical journals such as the Journal of the American Medical Association and New England Journal of Medicine.
Your library may also carry searchable computer databases of medical journal articles, including MEDLINE/PubMed or the Cumulative Index to Nursing and Allied Health Literature. Many of the databases or indexes have abstracts that provide a summary of each journal article. Although most community libraries don't have a large collection of medical and nursing journals, your librarian may be able to get copies of the articles you want. Interlibrary loans allow your librarian to request a copy of an article from a library that carries that particular medical journal. Your library may charge a fee for this service. Articles published in medical journals can be technical, but they may be the most current source of information on medical topics.

44. What is the main idea of the passage?
    a. Infotrac is a useful source of information.
    b. The community library offers numerous resources for medical information.
    c. Searching for medical information can be confusing.
    d. There is no reason to prepare a list of topics before visiting the library.

45. What is the meaning of the word *popular* as it is used in the third paragraph?
    a. complicated
    b. old-fashioned
    c. beloved
    d. for the general public

46. Which statement is *not* a detail from the passage?
    a. Abstracts summarize the information in an article.
    b. Having a prepared list of questions enables the librarian to serve you better.
    c. Infotrac is a database on CD-ROM.
    d. The articles in popular magazines can be hard to understand.

47. What is the meaning of the word *technical* as it is used in the fourth paragraph?
    a. requiring expert knowledge
    b. incomplete
    c. foreign
    d. plagiarized

Reading Comprehension Answer Key and Explanations

1. D: The main idea of this passage is that vaccines help the immune system function properly. Identifying main ideas is one of the key skills tested by the HESI exam. One of the common traps that many test-takers fall into is assuming that the first sentence of the passage will express the main idea. Although this will be true for some passages, often the author will use the first sentence to attract interest or to make an introductory, but not central, point. On this question, if you assume that the first sentence contains the main idea, you will mistakenly choose answer B. Finding the main idea of a passage requires patience and thoroughness; you cannot expect to know the main idea until you have read the entire passage. In this case, a diligent reading will show you that answer choices A, B, and C express details from the passage, but only answer choice D is a comprehensive summary of the author's message.

2. C: This passage does not state that the symptoms of disease will not emerge until the body has learned to fight the disease. The reading comprehension section of the HESI exam will include several questions that require you to identify details from a passage. The typical structure of these questions is to ask you to identify the answer choice that contains a detail not included in the passage. This question structure makes your work a little more difficult, because it requires you to confirm that the other three details are in the passage. In this question, the details expressed in answer choices A, B, and D are all explicit in the passage. The passage never states, however, that the symptoms of disease do not emerge until the body has learned how to fight the disease-causing microbe. On the contrary, the passage implies that a person may become quite sick and even die before the body learns to effectively fight the disease.

3. B: In the third paragraph, the word *virulent* means "malicious." The reading comprehension section of the HESI exam will include several questions that require you to define a word as it is used in the passage. Sometimes the word will be one of those used in the vocabulary section of the exam; other times, the word in question will be a slightly difficult word used regularly in academic and professional circles. In

some cases, you may already know the basic definition of the word. Nevertheless, you should always go back and look at the way the word is used in the passage. The HESI exam will often include answer choices that are legitimate definitions for the given word, but which do not express how the word is used in the passage. For instance, the word *virulent* could in some circumstances mean contagious or annoying. However, since the passage is not talking about transfer of the disease and is referring to a serious illness, malicious is the more appropriate answer.

4. C: The author's primary purpose in writing this essay is to inform. The reading comprehension section of the HESI exam will include a few questions that ask you to determine the purpose of the author. The answer choices are always the same: The author's purpose is to entertain, to persuade, to inform, or to analyze. When an author is *writing to entertain*, he or she is not including a great deal of factual information; instead, the focus is on vivid language and interesting stories. *Writing to persuade* means "trying to convince the reader of something." When a writer is just trying to provide the reader with information, without any particular bias, he or she is *writing to inform*. Finally, *writing to analyze* means to consider a subject already well known to the reader. For instance, if the above passage took an objective look at the pros and cons of various approaches to fighting disease, we would say that the passage was a piece of analysis. Because the purpose of this passage is to present new information to the reader in an objective manner, however, it is clear that the author's intention is to inform.

5. A: The subject of this passage is foodborne illnesses. Identifying the subject of a passage is similar to identifying the main idea. Do not assume that the first sentence of the passage will declare the subject. Oftentimes, an author will approach his or her subject by first describing some related, familiar subject. In this passage, the author does introduce the subject of the passage in the first sentence. However, it is only by reading the rest of the passage that you can determine the subject. One way to figure out the subject of a passage is to identify the main idea of each paragraph, and then identify the common thread in each.

6. B: This passage never states that cooked food cannot cause illness. Indeed, the first sentence of the third paragraph states that harmful bacteria can be present on cooked food that is left out for two or more hours. This is a direct contradiction of answer choice B. If you can identify an answer choice that is clearly contradicted by the text, you can be sure that it is not one of the ideas advanced by the passage. Sometimes the correct answer to this type of question will be something that is contradicted in the text; on other occasions, the correct answer will be a detail that is not included in the passage at all.

7. C: In the first paragraph, the word *pathogens* means "disease-causing substances." The vocabulary you are asked to identify in the reading comprehension section of the HESI exam will tend to be health related. The exam administrators are especially interested in your knowledge of the terminology used by doctors and nurses. Some of these words, however, are rarely used in normal conversation, so they may be unfamiliar to you. The best way to determine the meaning of an unfamiliar word is to examine how it is used in context. In the last sentence of the first paragraph, it is clear that pathogens are some substances that cause disease. Note that the pathogens are not diseases themselves; we would not say that an uncooked piece of meat "has a disease," but rather that consuming it "can cause a disease." For this reason, answer choice C is better than answer choice A.

8. A: In the second paragraph, the word *sterile* means "free of bacteria." This question provides a good example of why you should always refer to the word as it is used in the text. The word *sterile* is often used to describe "a person who cannot reproduce." If this definition immediately came to mind when you read the question, you might have mistakenly chosen answer D. However, in this passage the author describes raw foods as *not sterile*, meaning that they contain bacteria. For this reason, answer choice A is the correct response.

9. C: The main idea of the passage is that both the esophagus and the stomach are subject to bleeding problems. The structure of this passage is simple: The first paragraph discusses bleeding disorders of the esophagus, and the second paragraph discusses bleeding disorders of the stomach. Remember that statements can be true, and can even be explicitly stated in the passage, and can yet not be the main idea of the passage. The main idea given in answer choice A is perhaps true, but is too general to be classified as the main idea of the passage.

10. B: The passage never states that ulcer disease rarely occurs in the stomach. On the contrary, in the second paragraph the author states that ulcer disease *can* affect the blood vessels in the stomach. The three other answer choices can be found within the passage. The surest way to answer a question like this is to comb through the passage, looking for each detail in turn. This is a time-consuming process, however, so you may want to follow any initial intuition you have. In other words, if you are suspicious of one of the answer choices, see if you can find it in the passage. Often you will find that the detail is expressly contradicted by the author, in which case you can be sure that this is the right answer.

11. A: In the first paragraph, the word *rupture* means "tear." All of the answer choices are action verbs that suggest destruction. In order to determine the precise meaning of rupture, then, you must examine its usage in the passage. The author is describing a condition in which damage to a vein causes internal bleeding. Therefore, it does not make sense to say that the vein has *collapsed* or *imploded*, as neither of these verbs suggests a ripping or opening in the side of the vein. Similarly, the word *detach* suggests an action that seems inappropriate for a vein. It seems quite possible, however, for a vein to *tear*: Answer choice A is correct.

12. D: In the second paragraph, the word *erode* means "wear away." Your approach to this question should be the same as for question 11. Take a look at how the word is used in the passage. The author is describing a condition in which ulcers degrade a vein to the point of bleeding. Obviously, it is not appropriate to say that the ulcer has *avoided*, *divorced*, or *contained* the vein. It *is* sensible, however, to say that the ulcer has *worn away* the vein.

13. A: The primary subject of the passage is a new artificial retina. This question is a little tricky, because the author spends so much time talking about the experience of Kathy Blake. As a reader, however, you have to ask yourself whether Mrs. Blake or the new artificial retina is more essential to the story. Would the author still be interested in the story if a different person had the artificial retina? Probably. Would the author have written about Mrs. Blake if she hadn't gotten the artificial retina? Almost certainly not. Really, the story of Kathy Blake is just a way for the author to make the artificial retina more interesting to the reader. Therefore, the artificial retina is the primary subject of the passage.

14. B: In the second paragraph, the word *progressive* means "gradually increasing." The root of the word is *progress*, which you may know means "advancement toward a goal." With this in mind, you may be reasonably certain that answer choice B is correct. It is never a bad idea to examine the context, however. The author is describing *progressive visual loss*, so you might be tempted to select answer choice C or D, since they both suggest loss or diminution. Remember, however, that the adjective *progressive* is modifying the noun *loss*. Since the *loss* is increasing, the correct answer is B.

15. C: The passage never states that retinitis pigmentosa (RP) is curable. This question may be somewhat confusing, since the passage discusses a new treatment for RP. However, the passage never declares that researchers have come up with a cure for the condition; rather, they have developed a new technology that allows people who suffer from RP to regain some of their vision. This is not the same thing as curing RP. Kathy Blake and others like her still have RP, though they have been assisted by this exciting new technology.

16. D: The author's intention in writing this essay is to inform. You may be tempted to answer that the author's intention is to entertain. Indeed, the author expresses his message through the story of Kathy Blake. This story, however, is not important by itself. It is clearly included as a way of explaining the new camera glasses. If the only thing the reader learned from the passage was the story of Kathy Blake, the author would probably be disappointed. At the same time, the author is not really trying to persuade the reader of anything. There is nothing controversial about these new glasses: Everyone is in favor of them. The mission of the author, then, is simply to inform the reader.

17. A: The main idea of the passage is that Usher syndrome is an inherited condition that affects hearing and vision. Always be aware that some answers may be included in the passage but not the main idea. In this question, answer choices B and D are both true details from the passage, but neither of them would be a good summary of the article. One way to approach this kind of question is to consider what you would be likely to say if someone asked you to describe the article in a single sentence. Often, the sentence you come up with will closely mimic one of the answer choices. If so, you can be sure that answer choice is correct.

18. D: In the first paragraph, the word *symptoms* means "perceptible signs." The word *symptoms* is used frequently in medical contexts, though many people do not entirely understand its meaning. Symptoms are only those signs of illness that can be observed by someone besides the person with the illness. A stomachache, for instance, is not technically considered a symptom, since it cannot be observed by anyone other than the person who has it. A rash, however, is considered a symptom because other people can see it. The best definition for *symptoms*, then, is perceptible signs; that is, signs that can be perceived.

19. B: The passage does not state that Usher syndrome affects both hearing and smell. On the contrary, the passage only states that Usher syndrome affects hearing and vision. You should not be content merely to note that sentence in the passage and select answer choice B. In order to be sure, you need to quickly scan the passage to determine whether there is any mention of problems with the sense of smell. This is because the mention of impaired hearing and vision does not make it impossible for smell to be damaged as well. It is a good idea to practice scanning short articles for specific words. In this case, you would want to scan the article looking for words like *smell* and *nose*.

20. C: In the second paragraph, the word *juvenile* means "occurring in children." Examine the context in which the word is used. Remember that the context extends beyond just the immediate sentence in which the word is found. It can also include adjacent sentences and paragraphs. In this case, the word juvenile is immediately followed by a further explanation of Usher syndrome as it appears in children. You can be reasonably certain, then, that juvenile Usher syndrome is the condition as it presents in children. Although the word *juvenile* is occasionally used in English to describe immature or annoying behavior, it is clear that the author is not here referring to a *bratty* form of Usher syndrome.

21. B: In the third paragraph, the word *mutated* means "altered." This word comes from the same root as mutant; a *mutant* is an organism in which the chromosomes have been changed somehow. The context in which the word is used makes it clear that the author is referring to a scenario in which one of the parent's chromosomes has been altered. One way to approach this kind of problem is to substitute the answer choice into the passage to see if it still makes sense. Clearly, it would not make sense for a chromosome to be *selected*, since chromosomes are passed on and inherited without conscious choice. Neither does it make sense for a chromosome to be destroyed, because a basic fact of biology is that all living organisms have chromosomes.

22. D: The main idea of the passage is that the immune system protects the body from infection. The author repeatedly alludes to the complexity and mystery of the immune system, so it cannot be true that scientists fully understand this part of the body. It is true that the immune system triggers the production

- 105 -

of fluids, but this description misses the point. Similarly, it is true that the body is under constant invasion by malicious microbes; however, the author is much more interested in the body's response to these microbes. For this reason, the best answer choice is D.

23. C: The passage never states that viruses are extremely sophisticated. In fact, the passage explicitly states the opposite. However, in order to know this you need to understand the word *primitive*. The passage says that viruses are too primitive, or early in their development, to be classified as living organisms. A primitive organism is simple and undeveloped—exactly the opposite of sophisticated. If you do not know the word *primitive*, you can still answer the question by finding all three of the answer choices in the passage.

24. D: In the first paragraph, the word *ideal* means "perfect." Do not be confused by the similarity of the word *ideal* to *idea* and mistakenly select answer choice A. Take a look at the context in which the word is used. The author is describing how many millions of microbes can live inside the human body. It would not make sense, then, for the author to be describing the body as a *hostile* environment for microbes. Moreover, whether or not the body is a confined environment would not seem to have much bearing on whether it is good for microbes. Rather, the paragraph suggests that the human body is a perfect environment for microbes.

25. B: The passage never states that the immune system ignores tumors. Indeed, at the beginning of the third paragraph, the author states that scientists remain puzzled by the body's ability to fight tumors. This question is a little tricky, because it is common knowledge that many tumors prove fatal to the human body. However, you should not take this to mean that the body does not at least try to fight tumors. In general, it is best to seek out direct evidence in the text rather than to rely on what you already know. You will have enough time on the HESI exam to fully examine and research each question.

26. A: In the second paragraph, the word *enlist* means "call into service." The use of this word is an example of figurative language, the use of a known image or idea to elucidate an idea that is perhaps unfamiliar to the reader. In this case, the author is describing the efforts of the immune system as if they were a military campaign. The immune system *enlists* other cells, and then directs these *recruits* to areas where they are needed. You are probably familiar with *enlistment* and *recruitment* as they relate to describe military service. The author is trying to draw a parallel between the enlistment of young men and women and the enlistment of immune cells. For this reason, "call into service" is the best definition for *enlist*.

27. C: The author's primary purpose in writing this essay is to inform. As you may have noticed, the essays included in the reading comprehension section of the HESI exam were most often written to inform. This should not be too surprising; after all, the most common intention of any writing on general medical subjects is to provide information rather than to persuade, entertain, or analyze. This does not mean that you can automatically assume that "to inform" will be the answer for every question of this type. However, if you are in doubt, it is probably best to select this answer. In this case, the passage is written in a clear, declarative style with no obvious prejudice on the part of the author. The primary intention of the passage seems to be providing information about the immune system to a general audience.

28. B: The main idea of the passage is that the Food and Drug Administration (FDA) has a special program for regulating dietary supplements. This passage has a straightforward structure: The author introduces his subject in the first paragraph and uses the four succeeding paragraphs to elaborate. All of the other possible answers are true statements from the passage but cannot be considered the main idea. One way to approach questions about the main idea is to take sentences at random from the passage and see which answer choice they could potentially support. The main idea should be strengthened or supported by most of the details from the passage.

29. D: The passage never states that the Food and Drug Administration (FDA) ignores products after they enter the market. In fact, the entire fourth paragraph describes the steps taken by the FDA to regulate products once they are available for purchase. In some cases, questions of this type will contain answer choices that are directly contradictory. Here, for instance, answer choices A and B cannot be true if answer choice D is true. If there are at least two answer choices that contradict another answer choice, it is a safe bet that the contradicted answer choice cannot be correct. If you are at all uncertain about your logic, however, you should refer to the passage.

30. C: In the third paragraph, the phrase *phased in* means "implemented in stages." Do not be tempted by the similarity of this phrase to the word *fazed*, which can mean "confused or stunned." The author is referring to manufacturing standards that have already been implemented for large manufacturers and are in the process of being implemented for small manufacturers. It would make sense, then, for these standards to be implemented in *phases*: that is, to be *phased in*.

31. A: In the fifth paragraph, the word *deceptive* means "misleading." The root of the word *deceptive* is the same as for the words *deceive* and *deception*. Take a look at the context in which the word is used. The author states that the FDA prevents certain kinds of advertising. It would be somewhat redundant for the author to mean that the FDA prevents *illegal* advertising; this goes without saying. At the same time, it is unlikely that the FDA spends its time trying to prevent merely *irritating* advertising; the persistent presence of such advertising makes this answer choice inappropriate. Left with a choice between *malicious* and *misleading* advertising, it makes better sense to choose the latter, since being mean and nasty would be a bad technique for selling a product. It is common, however, for an advertiser to deliberately mislead the consumer.

32. B: The main idea of the passage is that anemia is a potentially dangerous condition characterized by low numbers of RBCs (red blood cells). All of the other answer choices are true (although answer C leaves out RBCs), but only answer choice C expresses an idea that is supported by the others. When you are considering a question of this type, try to imagine the answer choices as they would appear on an outline. If the passage above were placed into outline form, which answer choice would be the most appropriate title? Which answer choices would be more appropriate as supporting details? Try to get in the habit of imagining a loose outline as you are reading the passages on the HESI exam.

33. D: The passage never states that anemia is rarely caused by blood loss. On the contrary, in the first sentence of the fourth paragraph the author lists three causes of anemia, and blood loss is listed first. Sometimes, answer choices for this type of question will refer to details not explicitly mentioned in the passage. For instance, answer choice A is true without ever being stated in precisely those terms. Since the passage mentions several different treatments for anemia, however, you should consider the detail in answer choice A to be in the passage. In other words, it is not enough to scan the passage looking for an exact version of the detail. Sometimes, you will have to use your best judgment.

34. D: In the third paragraph, the word *oxygenated* means "containing high amounts of oxygen." This word is not in common usage, so it is absolutely essential for you to refer to its context in the passage. The author states in the second paragraph that anemia is in part a deficiency of the red blood cells that carry oxygen throughout the body. Then in the first sentence of the third paragraph, the author states that anemic individuals do not get enough oxygenated blood. Given this information, it is clear that *oxygenated* must mean carrying high amounts of oxygen, because it has already been stated that anemia consists of a lack of oxygen-rich blood.

35. A: In the fifth paragraph, the word *severity* means "seriousness." This word shares a root with the word *severe*, but not with the word *sever*. As always, take a look at the word as it is used in the passage. In

- 107 -

the final sentence of the passage, the author states that the treatment for anemia will depend on the *cause and severity* of the condition. In the previous paragraph, the author outlined a treatment for anemia and indicated that the proper response to the condition varies. The author even refers to the worst cases of anemia as being *severe*. With this in mind, it makes the most sense to define *severity* as seriousness.

36. C: The main idea of the passage is that a recent study found no link between caffeine consumption and rheumatoid arthritis (RA) among women. As is often the case, the first sentence of the passage contains the main idea. However, do not assume that this will always be the case. Furthermore, do not assume that the first sentence of the passage will only contain the main idea. In this passage, for instance, the author makes an immediate reference to the previous belief in the correlation between caffeine and RA. It would be incorrect, however, to think that this means answer choice A is correct. Regardless of whether or not the main idea is contained in the first sentence of the passage, you will need to read the entire text before you can be sure.

37. A: The passage never states that alcohol consumption is linked with RA. The passage does state that the new study took into account alcohol consumption when evaluating the long-term data. This is a good example of a question that requires you to spend a little bit of time rereading the passage. A quick glance might lead you to believe that the new study had found a link between alcohol and RA. Tricky questions like this make it even more crucial for you to go back and verify each answer choice in the text. Working through this question by using the process of elimination is the best way to ensure the correct response.

38. A: In the second paragraph, the word *symmetrical* means "affecting both sides of the body in corresponding fashion." This is an example of a question that is hard to answer even after reviewing its context in the passage. If you have no idea what *symmetrical* means, it will be hard for you to select an answer: All of them sound plausible. In such a case, the best thing you can do is make an educated guess. One clue is that the author has been describing a condition that affects the hands and the feet. Since people have both right and left hands and feet, it makes sense that inflammation would be described as *symmetrical* if it affects both the right and left hand or foot.

39. B: The author's primary purpose in writing this essay is to inform. You may be tempted to select answer choice D on the grounds that the author is presenting a particular point of view. However, there is no indication that the author is trying to persuade the reader of anything. One clear sign that an essay is written to persuade is a reference to what the reader already thinks. A persuasive essay assumes a particular viewpoint held by the reader and then argues against that viewpoint. In this passage, the author has no allegiance to any idea; he or she is only reporting the results of the newest research.

40. C: The main idea of the passage is that exercise improves bone health. This short passage has a simple structure: The author presents the thesis (main idea) and then spends the rest of the essay supporting it. When a passage is as clearly organized as this one, there should be little mystery about the main idea. If you look at the first sentences of paragraphs two and three, you will see that both contain the words *exercise* and *bones*. This is a good sign that either answer choice A or C is correct. Once you note that weight-bearing exercise is not discussed until the final paragraph, it seems clear that the correct answer must be C.

41. B: In the first paragraph, the word *vital* means "important." On first looking at this word, you might note its similarity to other words having to do with life and liveliness: *vitality*, *revive*, and *vivacious*, to name just a few. This knowledge can help guide your response, though you shouldn't make any assumptions based on it. Otherwise, you might mistakenly select answer choice D. The author states that exercise is *vital* for healthy bones. It would not make sense to say that exercise is *nourishing* for healthy bones, because it would also be so for unhealthy bones. The author is not describing the condition of

healthy bones, but rather how bones can be made healthy. For this reason, it makes the most sense to select answer choice B.

42. C: The passage never states that swimming is not good for the bones. This question is a little bit tricky, because the author does state that non-weight-bearing forms of exercise, including swimming, are not *as* good for the bones as weight-bearing exercises. However, just because swimming is not as good for the bones as running does not mean that it is bad for the bones. In fact, swimming works every major muscle system of the body and contributes to overall health, which includes bone health. Be on guard for questions like this that try to fool you into putting words in the author's mouth.

43. A: In the second paragraph, the word *fractures* means "breaks." In the second paragraph, the author declares that exercise reduces the risk of falls and fractures. To begin with, it makes sense to assume that broken bones would be one of the possible results of a fall. We are all aware that older people are more likely to break their bones by falling in the shower or on the stairs. On occasion, authors will use the word *fracture* to describe a damaged relationship, which may tempt you to select *tiffs*. In this case, however, the context makes clear that the author is describing broken bones.

44. B: The main idea of the passage is that the community library offers numerous resources for medical information. While most of the articles used in the reading comprehension section of the HESI exam will be about scientific or health-related concepts directly, some will touch on health and medicine in a more indirect manner. In this article, the author outlines some of the useful sources of medical information that can be obtained at the local library. Answer choices A and C are true, but do not express the general, overarching message of the article. Answer choice D is not true and is directly contradicted by the article itself.

45. D: In the third paragraph, the word *popular* means "for the general public." This word is more often used to describe someone or something that is well known or liked, so you might be tempted to select answer choice C. Take a look at the word as it is used in the context of the third paragraph, however. The author states that the library contains popular magazines and newspapers and then adds that the library also contains medical journals. Popular magazines and newspapers, then, are not the same thing as professional trade journals. Because the latter are known to be complicated and technical (that is, requiring professional expertise), you can guess that *popular* magazines are for a general reading audience.

46. D: The passage does not state that the articles in popular magazines can be hard to understand. If you are working in order, you can use your knowledge of the word *popular* to figure out the answer to this question. Specifically, you will know that the word describes publications that are written for a general, nonexpert audience. With this in mind, it seems unlikely that the articles would also be hard to understand. The other three details are explicit in the passage, so the answer must be D.

47. A: In the fourth paragraph, the word *technical* means "requiring expert knowledge." Again, some of the details gleaned from your work in the preceding questions can help you. The word *technical* is used to describe medical journals. As has already been shown, the author states that medical journals are written for an expert audience and can be difficult for a nonprofessional to understand. If this is the case, you can infer that the word *technical* must mean requiring expert knowledge, answer choice A.

Vocabulary and General Knowledge Questions

1. What is the meaning of the word *prognosis*?
   a. forecast
   b. description
   c. outline
   d. schedule

2. What is the name for any substance that stimulates the production of antibodies?
   a. collagen
   b. hemoglobin
   c. lymph
   d. antigen

3. What is the best definition for the word *abstain*?
   a. offend
   b. retrain
   c. to refrain from
   d. defenestrate

4. Select the meaning of the underlined word in this sentence:
Jerry held out hope for recovery, in spite of the <u>ominous</u> results from the lab.
   a. threatening
   b. emboldening
   c. destructive
   d. insightful

5. What is the meaning of the word *incidence*?
   a. random events
   b. sterility
   c. autonomy
   d. rate of occurrence

6. Select the word that means "water loving."
   a. homologous
   b. hydrophilia
   c. dipsomaniac
   d. hydrated

7. Select the meaning of the underlined word in this sentence:
The <u>occluded</u> artery posed a significant threat to the long-term health of the patient.
   a. closed
   b. deformed
   c. enlarged
   d. engorged

8. What is the best description for the word *potent*?
   a. frantic
   b. determined
   c. feverish
   d. powerful

9. Select the meaning of the underlined word in this sentence:
The doctors were less concerned with Bill's respiration than with the <u>precipitous</u> rise in his blood pressure.
   a. detached
   b. sordid
   c. encompassed
   d. steep

10. Select the meaning of the underlined word in this sentence:
It is <u>vital</u> for the victim of a serious accident to receive medical attention immediately.
   a. recommended
   b. discouraged
   c. essential
   d. sufficient

11. What is the best description for the word *insidious*?
   a. stealthy
   b. deadly
   c. collapsed
   d. new

12. Select the word that means "take into the body."
   a. congest
   b. ingest
   c. collect
   d. suppress

13. What is the meaning of the word *proscribe*?
   a. anticipate
   b. prevent
   c. defeat
   d. forbid

14. Select the meaning of the underlined word in this sentence.
Wracked by abdominal pain, the victim of food poisoning moaned and rubbed his <u>distended</u> belly.
   a. concave
   b. sore
   c. swollen
   d. empty

15. Select the meaning of the underlined word in this sentence:
Despite the absence of <u>overt</u> signs, Dr. Harris suspected that Alicia might be suffering from the flu.
    a. concealed
    b. apparent
    c. expert
    d. delectable

16. Select the word that means "something added to resolve a deficiency or obtain completion."
    a. supplement
    b. complement
    c. detriment
    d. acumen

17. Select the word that means "a violent seizure."
    a. revelation
    b. nutrient
    c. contraption
    d. paroxysm

18. What is the meaning of *carnivore*?
    a. hungry
    b. meat eating
    c. infected
    d. demented

19. What is the meaning of *belligerent*?
    a. retired
    b. sardonic
    c. pugnacious
    d. acclimated

20. Select the word that means "on both sides."
    a. bilateral
    b. insufficient
    c. bicuspid
    d. congruent

21. Select the meaning of the underlined word in this sentence:
The medication should only be taken if the old symptoms <u>recur</u>.
    a. occur again
    b. survive
    c. collect
    d. desist

22. Select the word that means "likely to change."
    a. venereal
    b. motile
    c. labile
    d. entrail

23. What is the best description for the word *flaccid*?
    a. defended
    b. limp
    c. slender
    d. outdated

24. Select the word that means "both male and female."
    a. monozygotic
    b. heterogeneous
    c. homologous
    d. androgynous

25. What is the meaning of *terrestrial*?
    a. alien
    b. earthly
    c. foreign
    d. domestic

26. Select the word that means "improper or unfortunate."
    a. allocated
    b. untoward
    c. flaccid
    d. dilated

27. Select the meaning of the underlined word in this sentence:
At first, Gerald suspected that he had caught the disease at the office; later, though, he concluded that it was underlined endogenous.
    a. contagious
    b. painful to the touch
    c. continuous
    d. growing from within

28. What is the meaning of *symptom*?
    a. result
    b. indication
    c. side effect
    d. precondition

29. Select the word that means "intrusive."
    a. convulsive
    b. destructive
    c. invasive
    d. connective

30. What is the meaning of *parameter*?
    a. guideline
    b. standard
    c. manual
    d. variable

31. Select the word that means "empty."
    a. holistic
    b. void
    c. concrete
    d. maladjusted

32. Select the meaning of the underlined word in this sentence:
Though chemotherapy had sent her cancer into remission, Glenda remained <u>lethargic</u> and depressed.
    a. nauseous
    b. sluggish
    c. contagious
    d. elated

33. Select the word that means "offsetting."
    a. compensatory
    b. defensive
    c. untoward
    d. confused

34. Select the word that means "degeneration or wasting away."
    a. dystrophy
    b. entropy
    c. atrophy
    d. apathy

35. What is the best description for the word *discrete*?
    a. calm
    b. subtle
    c. hidden
    d. separate

36. Select the meaning of the underlined word in this sentence:
In order to minimize scarring, the nurse reused the <u>site</u> of the previous injection.
    a. syringe
    b. location
    c. artery
    d. hole

37. Select the meaning of the underlined word in this sentence:
As a veteran of many flu seasons, the nurse knew how to minimize her <u>exposure</u> to the disease.
    a. laying open
    b. prohibition
    c. connection
    d. dislike

38. What is the meaning of *exacerbate*?
    a. implicate
    b. aggravate
    c. heal
    d. decondition

39. Select the word that means "nerve cell."
   a. neutron
   b. nucleus
   c. neuron
   d. neutral

40. Select the word that means "unfavorable."
   a. liberated
   b. adverse
   c. convenient
   d. occluded

41. Select the meaning of the underlined word in this sentence:
Dr. Grant ignored Mary's particular symptoms, instead administering a <u>holistic</u> treatment for her condition.
   a. insensitive
   b. ignorant
   c. specialized
   d. concerned with the whole rather than the parts

42. What is the best description for the word *suppress*?
   a. stop
   b. push up
   c. release
   d. strain

43. Select the word that means "about to happen."
   a. depending
   b. offending
   c. suspending
   d. impending

44. Select the meaning of the underlined word in this sentence:
The dermatologist was struck by the <u>symmetric</u> patterns of scarring on the patient's back.
   a. scabbed
   b. painful to the touch
   c. occurring in corresponding parts at the same time
   d. geometric

45. Select the word that means "open."
   a. inverted
   b. patent
   c. convent
   d. converted

46. Select the meaning of the underlined word in this sentence:
Despite an increase in the <u>volume</u> of his urine, the patient still reported bloating.
   a. quality
   b. length
   c. quantity
   d. loudness

47. What is the meaning of *repugnant*?
    a. destructive
    b. selective
    c. collective
    d. offensive

48. Select the word that means "enlarge."
    a. dilate
    b. protrude
    c. confuse
    d. occlude

49. What is the best description for the word *intact*?
    a. collapsed
    b. disconnected
    c. unbroken
    d. free

50. Select the word that means "the ability to enter, contact, or approach."
    a. ingress
    b. excess
    c. access
    d. success

Vocabulary and General Knowledge Answer Key and Explanations

1. A: The best definition for the word *prognosis* is "forecast." A prognosis is a probable result or course of a disease. The prognosis usually includes the likelihood of recovery for the patient. A prognosis is distinct from a *diagnosis*, which is just the description of the patient's condition. Likewise, a *description* is not the same thing as a prognosis, because it does not include a suggestion of what will happen in the future. An *outline* is an organized description of a subject, and therefore is not similar to a prognosis. Finally, a *schedule* is a plan for the future, rather than a prediction.

2. D: The name for a substance that stimulates the production of antibodies is an *antigen*. An antigen is any substance perceived by the immune system as dangerous. When the body senses an antigen, it produces an antibody. *Collagen* is one of the components of bone, tendon, and cartilage. It is a spongy protein that can be turned into gelatin by boiling. *Hemoglobin* is the part of red blood cells that carries oxygen. In order for the blood to carry enough oxygen to the cells of the body, there has to be a sufficient amount of hemoglobin. *Lymph* is a near-transparent fluid that performs a number of functions in the body: It removes bacteria from tissues, replaces lymphocytes in the blood, and moves fat away from the small intestine. Lymph contains white blood cells. As you can see, some of the questions in the vocabulary section will require technical knowledge.

3. C: The best definition for the word *abstain* is "to refrain from." Doctors often ask their patients to abstain from certain behaviors that have a negative impact on health. For example, a patient recovering from a viral infection might be asked to abstain from alcohol, so as to prevent weakening of the immune system. To *offend* is "to annoy or irritate." A health-care worker should take care to avoid offending a patient. *Retrain* means "to teach someone how to do a job again." For instance, a nurse might have to be

retrained after a long period of not performing a particular task. To *defenestrate* means "to throw out the window." This word is unlikely to be used in a health context.

4. A: The best synonym for *ominous* as it is used in this sentence is "threatening." An ominous symptom, for instance, is one that suggests the presence of serious disease. The word *emboldening* means "making bold." A patient who is regaining strength might be emboldened to try new and more difficult activities. The word *destructive* means "causing damage, chaos, or loss." A destructive condition or behavior has a negative effect on the patient's health. The word *insightful* means "thoughtful or provocative." As a health practitioner, you should try to be insightful so that you can come up with creative solutions to your patients' problems.

5. D: The word *incidence* means "rate of occurrence." A doctor will often refer to the incidence of a particular disease or condition as a measure of its severity or longevity. *Random events* are referred to as "incidents." *Sterility* means "free of living bacteria and microorganisms." It is absolutely necessary for a medical environment to be sterile so that patients will not get infections. *Autonomy* means "self-control and self-determination." A health-care worker should try to promote the autonomy of the patient whenever possible, although autonomy should never be more important than health and well-being.

6. B: *Hydrophilia* means "water loving." One could say that humans have a hydrophilic body, because our bodies crave constant infusions of water. The word *homologous* means "corresponding or having the same relative position or structure." A *dipsomaniac* is a person who cannot resist alcoholic drinks. Dipsomania is a compulsion that must be treated with behavioral therapy or medications such as Antabuse, which causes a violent physical reaction to alcohol. The word *hydrated* means "full of water or sufficiently full of water." Patients need to be hydrated, and medical workers need to be hydrated while they are performing their duties.

7. A: The closest meaning for the word *occluded* as it is used in this sentence is "closed." Occluded means "blocked or obstructed." The word is commonly used to describe arteries that no longer allow the passage of blood. The word *deformed* means "misshapen or out of the normal shape." Any deformed body part is a cause for concern. The word *engorged* means "overfull, especially of blood or food." The organs of the body may become engorged when they are infected or diseased. *Enlarged* means "made larger."

8. D: The best definition for the word *potent* is "powerful." A strong drug may be referred to as potent. The ability of a man to reproduce is sometimes referred to as his potency. The word *frantic* means "frenzied or anxious." A medical worker should never be frantic when dealing with patients and should do his or her best to keep patients from becoming frantic. The word *determined* means "set on a particular path." Whenever possible, a health-care worker should try to ensure that patients are determined to take the necessary steps toward recovery and good health. The word *feverish* can mean either "having a high temperature" or "being worried and anxious." A feverish patient should be comforted and given plenty of fluids.

9. D: The word *precipitous* as it is used this sentence means "steep." Doctors will often refer to a precipitous change in blood pressure. In general, precipitous changes are dangerous to the health. The word *detached* means "unconnected or aloof." A common example is a detached retina, a condition in which part of the eye becomes disconnected, and vision is damaged. The word *sordid* means "dirty" or "vile." The word *encompassed* means "surrounded or entirely contained within." For instance, a doctor might describe a treatment protocol as encompassing all aspects of the patient's life.

10. C: The word *vital* as it is used this sentence means "essential." Medical workers will often refer to a patient's vital signs, meaning blood pressure, heart rate, and temperature. The word *recommended* means "preferred by some authority." The recommended course of treatment is the one outlined and prescribed

by a doctor. The word *discouraged* means "disappointed and doubtful of success." Health-care workers should try to prevent patients from becoming discouraged, since this can further diminish quality of life and chances of recovery. The word *sufficient* means "having enough to accomplish the necessary task." As an example, a doctor might inquire to make sure that a patient is receiving sufficient fluids or food.

11. A: The best definition of the word *insidious* is "stealthy." An insidious disease takes root and develops in the body slowly, so that by the time the patient is aware of it, the damage can be severe and even fatal. Cancer is the classic example of insidious disease, because it may take root in the body and develop for a long period without any perceptible signs or symptoms. An insidious disease may be *deadly*, but it is not necessarily so. The words *collapsed* and *new* have no innate relationship to the word *insidious*.

12. B: The word *ingest* means "take into the body." The rate at which a patient ingests food and fluids is important when establishing a treatment protocol. To *congest* is "to fill to excess or to overcrowd." Chest congestion is a common complaint, which may be rooted in serious or minor causes. To *collect* is "to gather together." A health-care worker needs to collect information on patients so as to serve them effectively. To *suppress* means "to hold down or hold back." Patients should be encouraged not to suppress any information during a medical examination; keeping important facts from the doctor or nurse can prevent effective treatment.

13. D: The word *proscribe* means "forbid." A doctor often will proscribe certain foods or behaviors if they would negatively impact patient health. To *anticipate* is "to expect ahead of time." A doctor tries to anticipate how a disease will progress or how a patient will respond to treatment, though it is impossible to do this all the time. To *prevent* is "to keep from happening." Health-care workers try to prevent accidents and mistakes from happening on the job. To *defeat* is "to achieve victory over." The primary goal of treatment is to defeat whatever conditions are adversely affecting the patient's health.

14. C: The word *distended* as it is used in this sentence means "swollen." Doctors will often refer to a distended abdomen, which accompanies gassiness or bloating. The word *concave* means "shaped like the inside of a bowl." Many structures of the human body, for instance the inside of the ear and the arch of the foot, are described as concave. A distended body part may be *sore*, but it is not necessarily so. A distended artery, for instance, may have no accompanying pain. Also, though a distended body part may be *empty*, this is not always the case. In cases of starvation, the stomach may become distended; however, other body parts may become distended from being full to excess.

15. B: The word *overt* as it is used in this sentence means "apparent." Overt signs are those that can be seen by someone other than the person who is experiencing them. A rash is an overt sign; a stomachache is not. The word *concealed* means "hidden." Concealed signs cannot be perceived with the senses; a rise in blood pressure, for instance, is a concealed sign of illness. The word *expert*, used as an adjective, means "knowledgeable about a particular subject." When dealing with an unfamiliar situation, for instance, a doctor might call in an expert practitioner. The word *delectable* means "tasty or delicious."

16. A: The word *supplement* means "something added to resolve a deficiency or obtain completion." A doctor might recommend a particular nutritional supplement to address a patient's needs. A *complement* completes something or makes it perfect. Doctors try to put together complementary treatments that will reinforce and support one another. The word *detriment* means "loss, damage, or injury." A patient should be dissuaded from behaviors that will work to their detriment. The word *acumen* means "expertise" or "special knowledge in some area." A health-care worker will develop acumen based on his or her professional experience.

17. D: The word *paroxysm* means "a violent seizure." A patient who is suffering from paroxysms needs to be stabilized and treated immediately. A *revelation* is "a sudden realization or flash of knowledge."

Sometimes, a doctor will puzzle over a case until he or she has a revelation and realizes what needs to be done. A *nutrient* is "something that provides nutrition, or sustenance, to the body." Tests may indicate that a patient needs more of a particular nutrient in order to improve his or her health. A *contraption* is "a mechanical device." Health-care workers must learn how to use all sorts of contraptions in order to perform their duties.

18. B: The word *carnivore* means "meat eating." A patient who is not a carnivore might be in danger of anemia (iron deficiency) or other malnutrition. On the other hand, excessive consumption of red meat can lead to heart disease and obesity. *Hungry* means "feeling hunger." The word *infected* means "contaminated by germs." An infected body part needs to be sterilized and treated immediately. The word *demented* means "crazy or insane," especially when this behavior is the result of the condition known as dementia. A demented individual may not be able to make health-related decisions.

19. C: The word *belligerent* means "pugnacious." *Pugnacious* means "ready to fight." Belligerent patients may be resistant to treatment and disdainful of the doctor's or nurse's authority. The word *retired* means "withdrawn from business." The word *sardonic* means "mocking or sneering." This word is unlikely to come up in a medical context, though a health-care worker should avoid being sardonic. The word *acclimated* means "used to or accustomed to." Often, it takes a while for patients to become acclimated to a course of treatment or to a new lifestyle imposed upon them by diminishing health.

20. A: The word *bilateral* means "on both sides." This word is typically used to describe conditions that afflict both sides of the body. For instance, a patient suffering from bilateral partial paralysis might have numbness in both his right and left arms. The word *insufficient* means "lacking in necessary qualities." A patient might have insufficient blood flow to a certain area, or an insufficient amount of a certain nutrient. A *bicuspid* is anything that ends in two points. Many teeth are referred to as bicuspids because of their shape. The word *congruent* means "agreeing or in complete accord."

21. A: The word *recur* as it is used in this sentence means "occur again." Doctors often refer to the recurrence of a disease or symptom. In some cases, the recurrence of a disease indicates that the treatment used in the past was ineffective. *Recur* has the same root as *occur*, with the prefix *re-*, meaning "back or again." To *survive* means "to remain alive." To *collect* means "to bring together into one place." To *desist* means "to cease or stop doing something." A doctor might advise a patient to desist from a certain behavior in order to improve his or her health.

22. C: The word *labile* means "likely to change." This word is often used as a synonym for unstable. Blood pressure that fluctuates rapidly may be described as labile. The word *venereal* is used to describe conditions that relate to sexual intercourse. Venereal disease, for instance, is acquired during sexual contact. Chlamydia, gonorrhea, and syphilis are all examples of venereal disease. The word *motile* means "moving or capable of moving." A doctor will often refer to a part of the body as motile when its movements have been compromised in the past. An *entrail* is one of the internal parts of an animal or human body. It most often refers to the intestines.

23. B: The best description for the word *flaccid* is "limp." A flaccid part of the body is lacking in muscle tone. The word *defended* means "driven danger away from." The word *slender* means "thin or skinny, but not to the extent of being unhealthy." In general, patients who are slender recover better from injury and illness than patients who are overweight or obese. The word *outdated* describes "something that has become irrelevant with age." As medical technology becomes increasingly sophisticated, much of the equipment that used to be essential has now become outdated.

24. D: The word *androgynous* means "both male and female." Some children are born with androgynous characteristics, and their sexuality may remain ambiguous (hard to determine) for their entire life.

Monozygotic means "derived from one fertilized egg." Identical twins are often referred to as monozygotic because they emerge from an individual zygote (fertilized egg). The word *exogenous* is used to describe "conditions that originate outside of the body." It is not to be confused with *heterogeneous*, which means "having different parts." *Homologous* means "corresponding or having the same relative position." A dog's body is said to be homologous to a cat's because their legs are in the same place.

25. B: The word *terrestrial* means "earthly." It can also be used to refer to things that are from the land rather than from the water. The word *alien*, when used as an adjective, describes "things that are unfamiliar or from an outside source." *Alien* does not only refer to creatures from outer space. A patient who has come down with a mystery ailment might try to identify some contact with alien substances. The word *foreign* is used to describe "people or things that are from some other area or country." In an area where medical procedures are being performed, foreign objects are usually forbidden. The word *domestic* is used to describe "things that are of the home or household."

26. B: The word *untoward* means "improper or unfortunate." Health-care workers should avoid untoward actions when dealing with their patients. This means acting according to the professional code of ethics. *Allocated* means "reserved for a particular purpose." For example, a patient may be put on a specific exercise regimen. The patient then needs to allocate a certain part of the day for this activity, so that it is sure to be done. *Flaccid* means "limp or lacking in muscle tone." If a patient is experiencing any degree of paralysis, the affected part of the body may be flaccid. *Dilated* means "expanded or made larger." The pupils of the eyes become dilated in the dark so that more light can enter the lens.

27. D: The word *endogenous* as it is used in this sentence means "growing from within." Doctors occasionally refer to endogenous cholesterol, which comes from inside the body rather than from the diet. *Contagious* means "capable of spreading from person to person." A person with a contagious disease needs to be kept away from other people. Often, diseases are only contagious for a limited time. *Continuous* means "proceeding on without stopping." If a patient is suffering from continuous back pain, for instance, he or she is experiencing the pain at all times.

28. B: The word *symptom* means "indication." A symptom is any subjective indication of disease. A symptom can be perceived only by the patient. Lower back pain, for instance, is a symptom, because it cannot be perceived by anyone else. Symptoms are distinct from signs, which are apparent to the patient and other people. Bleeding and high blood pressure are both signs. In medicine, an *indication* is "a sign or symptom that suggests a particular treatment." For example, some rashes are an indication for topical ointment. A *side effect*, on the other hand, is "any effect in addition to the intended effect." The term is often used to describe the unpleasant additional effects of treatment or medication. As an example: Side effects of chemotherapy are nausea and fatigue. A *precondition* is "something that must happen or be true before something else can happen." For example, when a patient has the flu, keeping liquids down is a precondition for trying to eat solid foods.

29. C: The word *invasive* means "intrusive." An invasive disease seeks to penetrate the body and cause damage. Strep throat, a bacterial infection, is an example of an invasive disease. The word *convulsive* means "afflicted by spasms or seizures." A patient who suffers from epilepsy or extreme fever may become convulsive. Convulsive patients need to be stabilized so that they don't hurt themselves. The word *destructive* is used to describe "things that cause damage, injury, or loss." Health-care workers try to steer patients away from destructive behaviors. The word *connective* is used to describe "structures that bring other things into contact." The connective tissues of the body include cartilage, ligaments, and tendons.

30. A: The word *parameter* means "guideline." A doctor will often lay out certain parameters at the beginning of treatment. These are not specific rules, but rather they are the general ideas that will inform

the entire course of treatment. Parameters are the boundaries of treatment. A *standard*, on the other hand, is "an established basis of comparison." A *manual* is "a book that explains how to perform a particular task." A *variable* is "something that changes." The amount of food a patient is given might be considered to be a variable, for example.

31. B: The word *void* means "empty." Doctors may refer to a patient's bowels as void when they do not contain any digested food matter. *Holistic* means "concerned with the whole of something rather than with the particular parts." Doctors try to put together a holistic treatment plan so that the patient's general level of health will be improved. *Concrete* is a building material, but the word is also used as an adjective to describe "things that are real, sturdy, and well established." Doctors try to establish concrete standards for measuring a patient's condition, rather than relying on general impressions. *Maladjusted* means "poorly accustomed or acclimated." Although it often takes time for a patient to adjust to a new treatment protocol, some patients will remain maladjusted and require a change in treatment.

32. B: The word *lethargic* as it is used in this sentence means "sluggish." Lethargy is a symptom of many forms of illness. It is also a side effect of chemotherapy. *Nauseous* means "sickened, or suffering from an upset stomach." Nausea is a common side effect of chemotherapy as well; it is just not the one described in this sentence. *Contagious* means "capable of spreading from person to person." Many viral and bacterial infections are contagious. *Elated* means "ecstatic," or "wildly happy." It is usually a good thing when a patient is elated, although manic-depressive patients may alternate between excessive elation and near-suicidal sadness.

33. A: The word *compensatory* means "offsetting." A patient may develop compensatory behaviors to make up for a developing health condition. *Defensive* means "protective" or "intending to repel an attack." Sometimes, patients will feel defensive in the presence of a health professional. *Untoward* means "unfavorable, improper, or unfortunate." Untoward events will inevitably occur during the course of treatment; it is the job of the staff to continue their work regardless. *Confused* means "perplexed or bewildered." Some patients, especially the very young or very old, may become confused during treatment. When confusion is identified, health-care workers should slow down and help the patient feel more comfortable.

34. C: The word *atrophy* means "degeneration or wasting away." Doctors often refer to muscle atrophy, which occurs when a patient is immobile for a long period. Physical therapy and massage are two common ways to prevent muscle atrophy when a patient cannot move because of injury or illness. *Dystrophy* is "weakening, degeneration, or abnormal growth of muscle." You may have heard of muscular dystrophy, a hereditary disease in which the muscles gradually lose their strength. *Entropy* is "the tendency toward chaos and disorder." This term is occasionally used in a medical context to describe a patient's tendency toward decline and decrease in function. It is the job of the health-care worker to fight against entropy. *Apathy* is "a lack of caring." Patients who are suffering from serious injury or illness, especially those who have a poor long-term prognosis, may descend into apathy. A health-care worker should try to use his or her influence to improve mood and combat apathy.

35. D: The best description for the word *discrete* is "separate." Discrete symptoms, for example, are those that do not have any connection to one another, though they spring from the same source. The word *subtle* is used to describe things that are "delicate or mysterious in their meaning or intent." Sometimes, the signs of disease will be subtle. Although today's health-care system has amazing technology for spotting the signs of disease, health-care workers still must be on the lookout for the subtle signs of disease.

36. B: The word *site* as it is used in this sentence means "location." Doctors will often refer to the site of an injection or a planned surgery. A *syringe* is "the device used to inject or withdraw fluid from the body."

Medical personnel who specialize in withdrawing blood from patients are called phlebotomists. An *artery* is "a blood vessel that carries blood away from the heart to nourish the rest of the body." Although the site to which the author is referring in this sentence is a *hole*, it will not always be so. For this reason, "hole" cannot be the best definition for *site*.

37. A: The word *exposure* as it is used in this sentence means "laying open." The most common usage of this term is in reference to the sun, although exposure to toxic chemicals is also a major health concern. A doctor will often ask a patient to limit his or her exposure to some environmental element. *Prohibition* is "the act of forbidding." Often, a doctor will place a prohibition on certain behaviors or foods if they are believed to adversely affect health. The words *connection* and *dislike* have no relation to exposure.

38. B: The word *exacerbate* means "aggravate." The first commandment of medical care is "do no harm," which essentially means do nothing to exacerbate the patient's illness or injury. Behaviors or foods that exacerbate the symptoms of illness or injury should be stopped immediately. To *implicate* is "to demonstrate involvement or assign blame." Often, during the examination period, a doctor or nurse will implicate seemingly unrelated behaviors in a patient's condition. Once a behavior has been implicated, the doctor and patient will work together to eliminate its negative effects on health. To *decondition* is "to weaken or diminish the conditioned response to a certain stimulus." Part of working in health care is helping people make positive choices. In part, this is accomplished by deconditioning them to stimuli that provoke a negative response.

39. C: The word *neuron* means "nerve cell." The human body has millions of neurons, with billions of connections between them. A *neutron* is "the part of an atom that has neither positive nor negative charge." Neutrons are located in the nucleus of the atom. The *nucleus* is "the central part of a cell or atom, around which the other parts cluster." The HESI exam requires you to know the names and functions of all the cell parts. *Neutral* means "not taking part in or not taking sides in a dispute." A neutral behavior or medication is one that has neither a positive nor a negative effect on health.

40. B: The word *adverse* means "unfavorable." Unhealthy behaviors have an adverse effect on well-being. *Liberated* means "freed." The general goal of health care is to liberate patients from the negative effects of illness or injury. *Convenient* means "easily accessible and available." When health care is convenient, patients are more likely to acquire it. Health-care workers should strive to make their services convenient for patients whenever possible. *Occluded* means "blocked or closed." Patients with a high level of cholesterol are at risk of developing occluded arteries. Another instance in which the term is used is when a patient is choking: In this case, the patient's airway is said to be occluded.

41. D: The word *holistic* as it is used in this sentence means "concerned with the whole rather than the parts." Doctors try to consider the patient's health from a holistic perspective; that is, they try to improve health in its entirety rather than to eliminate specific symptoms. The word *insensitive* means "not responsive." The word *ignorant* means "lacking knowledge." Health-care workers cannot be ignorant of the latest findings and information in their field. The word *specialized* means "adapted to or trained in a specific discipline or task." Because of the technological complexity of modern medical practice, most careers in health care are specialized.

42. A: The best description for the word *suppress* is "stop." Sometimes, a patient will suppress their symptoms if they are not psychologically ready to face illness. However, the suppression of illness tends to create other problems. Ultimately, it is better not to suppress illness, but to face it directly. To *strain* is "to work hard or overextend." This word is used in a couple of different ways in health care. A patient may be suffering from a specific muscle strain after excessive exercise or hyperextension. Also, a doctor may prohibit a patient from straining in his or her professional life if it is causing fatigue and making the patient vulnerable to disease.

43. D: The word *impending* means "about to happen." A doctor might refer to impending symptoms, which are the symptoms the patient is likely to start experiencing in the near future. *Depending* means "relying on or placing trust in." Because most patients have no medical expertise, they are depending on doctors and nurses to choose the appropriate course of action. *Offending* means "annoying or irritating." *Suspending* means "stopping for an undetermined period." If a treatment is not working, for instance, or if it is causing unforeseen negative side effects, then a doctor may suspend it until more information can be gathered.

44. C: The word *symmetric* as it is used in this sentence means "occurring in corresponding parts at the same time." Some illnesses will cause symmetric rashes, meaning that both the right and left sides of the body are afflicted with similarly shaped inflammation. The word *scabbed* means "covered with wounds." The word *geometric* is used to describe "things that resemble the classic geometric shapes, such as the circle, square, or triangle." On occasion, a doctor may use this word to describe the pattern of a wound or rash.

45. B: The word *patent* means "open." Doctors will describe an artery as patent when it allows a free flow of blood. Similarly, a patent airway allows for unrestricted breathing. *Inverted* means turned upside down or backwards. Sometimes, a patient will be inverted in order to stimulate blood flow to certain parts of the body. A *convent* is "a home for nuns or monks." This word has no relevance to health care, but it is included because the HESI exam will sometimes try to tempt you with answer choices that sound like the right answer. The word *converted* means "changed or altered." A patient may have his or her diet converted in order to meet the needs of a treatment protocol.

46. C: The word *volume* as it is used in this sentence means "quantity." Doctors will refer to an increase in the volume of urine or some other body product as an indication of health. Volume is calculated as length × width × height (or depth); it is a three-dimensional measure. *Length*, on the other hand, is "a two-dimensional measure of distance." *Quality* means "degree of excellence." Quantity can be measured in any kind of units. *Loudness* might be the right answer if *volume* were being used in a different way, as "the relative power of a sound." In this sentence, however, the word is not being used to describe a sound.

47. D: The word *repugnant* means "offensive, especially to the senses or the morals." For instance, a patient may find a certain kind of medicine repugnant, in which case the doctor must either figure out a way to disguise the taste or consider a different form of treatment. The word *destructive* means "causing damage, injury, or loss." Patients should be steered away from destructive behaviors. *Selective* means "choosy or capable of making a thoughtful choice." In general, it is good to be selective, although a patient who is too selective about his or her diet may develop a nutritional deficiency. *Collective* means "combined or grouped together to form a whole." Health care seeks to treat the collective symptoms of the patient, rather than to focus on specific problems.

48. A: The word *dilate* means "enlarge." Dilation is often expressed as measurement, typically in units of centimeters. For instance, when the body becomes hot, the arteries dilate and blood rushes to the extremities. To *protrude* means "to stick out." Sometimes when a patient breaks a bone severely, part of the bone will protrude from the skin. To *occlude* means "to close up or block." Airways and arteries are the most common parts of the body to become occluded. Either of these occlusions needs to be dealt with immediately before other treatment can be administered.

49. C: The best description for the word *intact* is "unbroken." The word can be used in a number of different contexts. For instance, if a patient presents with severe pain in his or her side, the doctor might worry about the possibility of a ruptured appendix. After an X-ray reveals no damage to the appendix, however, the doctor might say that the organ is intact.

- 123 -

50. C: The word *access* means the ability "to enter, contact, or approach." It is important for patients to have easy access to health-care services. If patients do not have convenient access to services, they will be less likely to take actions to improve health. *Ingress* is "entering or going in." In some cases, a doctor will have to perform tests to determine a disease's path of ingress to the body. *Excess* is "too much or an overabundance of something." In general, excess of any kind is bad for the health. Even excessive exercise can be detrimental to health. During an initial examination, the doctor will try to identify areas in which the patient needs attention. *Success* is "the attainment of goals, whether personal, emotional, professional, physical, or financial." Obviously, the success of the patient is the top priority for all health-care workers.

Grammar Questions

1. Which word is *not* spelled correctly in the context of the following sentence?
Dr. Vargas was surprised that the prescription had effected Ron's fatigue so dramatically.
    a. surprised
    b. prescription
    c. effected
    d. fatigue

2. Select the word that makes this sentence grammatically correct:
Is the new student coming out to lunch with ____?
    a. we
    b. our
    c. us
    d. they

3. Select the word or phrase that makes this sentence grammatically correct:
____ picking up groceries one of the things you are supposed to do?
    a. Is
    b. Am
    c. Is it
    d. Are

4. Select the word that makes the following sentence grammatically correct.
These days, you can't ____ learning how to use a computer.
    a. not
    b. evading
    c. despite
    d. avoid

5. Which word is *not* spelled correctly in the context of the following sentence?
The climate hear is inappropriate for snow sports such as skiing.
    a. climate
    b. hear
    c. inappropriate
    d. skiing

6. Select the word or phrase that makes the following sentence grammatically correct.
_____ screaming took the shopkeeper by surprise.
    a. We
    b. They
    c. Them
    d. Our

7. Select the word or phrase that makes the following sentence grammatically correct.
Why did we _____ try so hard?
    a. has to
    b. haven't
    c. had to
    d. have to

8. Select the word that makes the following sentence grammatically correct.
Tracey wore her hair in a French braid, _____ was the style at the time.
    a. among
    b. it
    c. that
    d. which

9. Select the phrase that makes the following sentence grammatically correct.
Working _____ the mission of the entire committee.
    a. to peace is
    b. toward peace was
    c. to peace was
    d. toward peace am

10. Select the phrase that makes the following sentence grammatically correct.
Janet called her _____ run after a squirrel.
    a. dog, who had
    b. dog that had
    c. dog, that had
    d. dog who had

11. Select the correct word for the blank in the following sentence.
After completing the intense surgery, Dr. Capra needed a long _____.
    a. brake
    b. break
    c. brink
    d. broke

12. Select the correct word for the blank in the following sentence.
The other day, Stan _____ reviewing his class notes in preparation for the final exam.
    a. begins
    b. begun
    c. begin
    d. began

13. Select the word or phrase that makes the following sentence grammatically correct.
It makes sense to maintain your current prescriptions, ____ they have worked so well in the past.
    a. although
    b. despite that
    c. since
    d. but

14. Select the word or phrase that makes the following sentence grammatically correct.
It seems like his blood pressure ___ every week.
    a. rises
    b. raises
    c. raise
    d. rise

15. Select the word or phrase that makes the following sentence correct.
____ their similar training, the two professionals drew radically different conclusions.
    a. Because of
    b. Among
    c. Despite
    d. Now that

16. Select the word or phrase that makes the following sentence grammatically correct.
Each of the two European capitals ____ named after a famous leader.
    a. are
    b. am
    c. as
    d. is

17. Which word is *not* used correctly in the context of the following sentence?
Before you walk any further, beware of the approaching traffic.
    a. before
    b. further
    c. beware
    d. approaching

18. What word is used incorrectly in the following sentence?
The little boy sat the red block atop the stack.
    a. little
    b. sat
    c. atop
    d. stack

19. Select the word or phrase that makes the following sentence grammatically correct.
Even though she was new, Lauren knew that ___ the patient's name would be an ethical violation.
    a. divulge
    b. to divulge
    c. to divulging
    d. divulged

20. Select the word or phrase that makes the following sentence grammatically correct.
The attendant looked _____ at everything related to the problem.
    a. close
    b. closet
    c. closely
    d. closedly

21. What word or phrase is used incorrectly in the following sentence?
Henry intuitively understood the doctor's illusion to his long-term depression.
    a. intuitively
    b. illusion
    c. long-term
    d. depression

22. Select the correct word for the blank in the following sentence.
If you want to join the club, you _____ contact the coach by Thursday.
    a. would
    b. should
    c. did
    d. have

23. Select the word that makes the following sentence grammatically correct.
Andy has _____ up a law practice of his own.
    a. seat
    b. set
    c. sit
    d. sat

24. Select the word or phrase that makes the following sentence grammatically correct.
He decided to buy a large coal furnace because he felt it would be _____ than a woodstove.
    a. more efficient
    b. efficienter
    c. more efficienter
    d. efficiency

25. What word is used incorrectly in the following sentence?
It is amazing how many soccer players has developed knee problems over the years.
    a. many
    b. players
    c. has
    d. developed

26. Select the word that makes the following sentence grammatically correct.
She asked ___ to take her around the corner to the drugstore.
    a. him
    b. his
    c. he
    d. his'

27. Select the word or phrase that makes the following sentence grammatically correct.
Felix was pleased _____ the progress he had made in his program.
  a. among
  b. with
  c. regards
  d. besides

28. Select the word or phrase that makes the following sentence grammatically correct.
After waking up, Dean eyed the cheesecake _____.
  a. hungry
  b. hungriest
  c. hungrily
  d. more hungry

29. Which word is *not* used correctly in the context of the following sentence?
After ringing up the nails, the cashier handed Nedra her recipe and change.
  a. ringing
  b. cashier
  c. recipe
  d. change

30. Select the correct word for the blank in the following sentence.
Sharon felt _____ about how her speech had gone.
  a. well
  b. good
  c. finely
  d. happily

31. What word is used incorrectly in the following sentence?
Brendan spent the day lying a brick foundation on the site.
  a. site
  b. on
  c. spent
  d. lying

32. Select the word or phrase that makes this sentence grammatically correct:
Children _____ obey their parents tend to do better in school.
  a. who
  b. which
  c. should
  d. to

33. Select the word or phrase that makes this sentence grammatically correct:
The development committee _____ a bargain with the city planners.
  a. striked
  b. stroke
  c. struck
  d. strike

- 128 -

34. Select the word or phrase that makes this sentence grammatically correct:
A child is not yet old enough to know what is healthy for _____.
    a. him or her
    b. them
    c. it
    d. she or he

35. Select the word or phrase that makes this sentence grammatically correct:
Theo was in great shape; he _____ all the way back to the pier.
    a. swam
    b. swimmed
    c. swum
    d. swim

36. Select the phrase that makes this sentence grammatically correct:
_____ went to the movies after having dinner at Lenny's.
    a. Her and I
    b. Her and me
    c. She and I
    d. She and me

37. Select the word or phrase that makes this sentence grammatically correct:
Before turning in, Brian made sure to ____ the alarm clock.
    a. sat
    b. sit
    c. set
    d. setted

38. What word is used incorrectly in the following sentence?
The dashboard shaked as he revved the engine.
    a. dashboard
    b. shaked
    c. as
    d. revved

39. Select the word or phrase that makes this sentence grammatically correct:
_____ way he looked, Ted saw people milling about.
    a. Moreover
    b. Whichever
    c. Whomever
    d. Whether

40. Select the correct word for the blank in the following sentence.
The buried treasure had ____ there for centuries.
    a. laid
    b. layed
    c. lain
    d. laint

41. Select the word that makes this sentence grammatically correct:
In order to serve each patient better, the clinic decided to see _____ patients overall.
   a. less
   b. fewer
   c. lesser
   d. few

42. Select the word or phrase that makes this sentence grammatically correct:
It wasn't until _____ the interview that Kim realized she had forgotten her list of questions.
   a. despite
   b. after
   c. among
   d. between

43. Which word is used incorrectly in the following sentence?
The video store is on the way, so we should stop by and rent one.
   a. video
   b. way
   c. by
   d. one

44. Select the word that makes the following sentence grammatically correct.
_____ are the best eye doctors in this county?
   a. Who
   b. Which
   c. Whom
   d. What

45. Select the word that makes this sentence grammatically correct:
While he was an apprentice, Steve _____ a great deal of time in the studio.
   a. spends
   b. spent
   c. spended
   d. spend

46. Select the word that correctly completes the following sentence.
The intern was surprised by the _____ of pain he was in after his first day of work.
   a. amount
   b. frequency
   c. number
   d. amplitude

47. What word is used incorrectly in the following sentence?
Whoever wrote the letter forgot to sign their name.
   a. Whoever
   b. wrote
   c. their
   d. name

48. Select the word or phrase that makes this sentence grammatically correct:
The child's fever was ___ high for him to lie comfortably in bed.
    a. to
    b. much
    c. too
    d. more

49. Select the word or phrase that makes the following sentence grammatically correct.
Sometimes, the condition _____ with an unusual symptom—vertigo.
    a. presence
    b. presents
    c. present
    d. prescience

50. Which word is *not* used correctly in the context of the following sentence?
There is no real distinction among the two treatment protocols recommended online.
    a. real
    b. among
    c. protocols
    d. online

Grammar Answer Key and Explanations

1. C: The word *effected* is not spelled correctly in the context of this sentence. In order to answer this question, you need to know the difference between *affect* and *effect*. The former is a verb and the latter is a noun. In other words, *affect* is something that you do and *effect* is something that is. In this sentence, the speaker is describing something that the prescription medication *did*. Therefore, the appropriate word is a verb. *Effect*, however, is a noun. For this reason, instead of *effected* the author should have used the word *affected*.

2. C: The word *us* makes the sentence grammatically correct. *Us* is the objective case of *we*. In this case, *us* is being used as an indirect object. An indirect object is the noun to which the action of the verb refers. In the sentence *He gave her a sandwich*, the indirect object is *her* (and the direct object is *sandwich*). All of the answer choices for this question are in the first-person plural, with the exception of answer choice D, which is in the third-person plural. The appropriate third-person plural form to complete this sentence is *them*.

3. A: The word *is* makes the sentence grammatically correct. In order to answer this question, you need to determine what the object of the verb will be. One way to do this is to rearrange the question as if it were a declarative sentence: *Picking up the groceries ____ one of the things you are supposed to do.* Expressed like this, it is easy to see that the subject of the sentence is "picking up the groceries." This is a third-person singular subject (that is, it is an "it"), so it receives the third-person present indicative verb form, *is*.

4. D: The word *avoid* makes the sentence grammatically correct. To *avoid* is to keep from doing something. The sentence states that it is impossible to function in the modern world without learning how to use a computer. The word *evade* has a similar meaning to *avoid*, but the verb form used here does not fit into the sentence correctly. The best way to approach this kind of question on the HESI exam is to read the sentence aloud softly, substituting in the various answer choices. If you used this strategy on question 4, you would immediately notice that answer choice B does not correctly complete the sentence.

5. B: The word *hear* is not spelled correctly in the context of this sentence. The speaker has mixed up the homophones *hear* and *here*. *Homophones* are words that sound the same but are spelled differently and have a different meaning. Homophones are not to be confused with *homonyms*, which are spelled the same but have a different meaning. In question 5, the author is trying to describe the place where the climate is; that is, he or she is describing the climate *here*. Unfortunately, the author uses the word *hear*, which is a verb meaning "to listen."

6. D: The word *our* makes the sentence grammatically correct. *Our* is the possessive case of *we*, In this case, our is being used as an attributive adjective. An adjective is a word that modifies (or describes) a noun. *Our* is called an attributive adjective because it is attributing (assigning) ownership of the screaming to a particular party, *us*. Answer choices A and D are in the first-person plural; answer choices B and C are in the third-person plural. Neither B nor C, however, is in the possessive case. The sentence could be effectively completed with *their*, but this choice is not available.

7. D: The phrase *have to* makes the sentence grammatically correct. The speaker is trying to express that his group was forced to try hard. For this reason, it is essential for the verb *have* to be used. *Have* is an auxiliary verb indicating obligation. It agrees with the first-person plural pronoun *we*. An auxiliary verb accompanies another verb and makes some alterations in mood or tense. In this case, the addition of the verb have indicates that the speaker and others were obliged to try hard. *Can*, *will*, and *have* are all common examples of auxiliary verbs.

8. D: The word *which* makes the sentence grammatically correct. In this sentence, *which* is used as a relative pronoun. A relative pronoun introduces a relative clause, which is so called because it "relates" to the antecedent. The antecedent is the word that the relative pronoun refers to. In this sentence, the antecedent is "French braid," and the subsequent relative clause gives the reader more information about the French braid. Answer choice C is also a relative pronoun, but it is rarely used after a comma.

9. B: The phrase *toward peace was* makes this sentence grammatically correct. The word *toward* is a preposition that can mean "in the direction of" or "with a view to obtaining." It is in this last sense that the word is being used in this sentence. Peace is an abstract concept, not a physical destination that one could actually reach. For this reason, it does not make sense to select answer choices A or C. Answer choice D has an incorrect verb form; since the subject of the sentence is "working toward peace," the third-person singular verb form is correct.

10. A: The phrase *dog, who had* makes the sentence grammatically correct. To begin with, it is necessary for there to be a comma separating these two clauses, because the second clause is nonrestrictive. A clause is considered nonrestrictive if it could not stand by itself and if the rest of the sentence would still make sense were it removed. If the portion of this sentence after the comma were removed, the sentence would be *Janet called her dog*. Obviously, this is still a coherent sentence. Also, *who* is used here instead of *which* because the antecedent, *dog*, has an identity and personality.

11. B: The word *break* correctly completes this sentence. This question hinges on the different meanings that can be assigned to the word *break*. A *break* can be a brief period of rest from work or some tiring activity, or it can be the act of destroying or disconnecting something. The first usage is as a noun, and the second usage is as a verb. In this sentence, the author is expressing that Dr. Capra needed something, which means you should use the noun form. Also, remember that a *brake* is the mechanism for stopping a vehicle.

12. D: The word *began* properly completes the sentence. The sentence begins with the phrase "the other day," which indicates that the action described took place sometime in the recent past. A past tense verb

- 132 -

form is appropriate, then. The verb *begun* is the past participle of *begin*. A past participle describes action that took place before but is now complete. This sentence does not indicate, however, that the action is now complete. For all we know, Stan could still be reviewing his class notes. For this reason, the past tense *began* is the correct answer.

13. C: The word *since* makes the sentence grammatically correct. In this sentence, *since* is being used as a conjunction meaning "because." The word can also be used as an adverb or a preposition indicating an interval from some past time to the present. In this sentence, however, the right answer is indicated by the context. The first part of the sentence states that the current prescription is to be maintained; this suggests that the speaker has a positive attitude toward it. It makes sense, then, that the prescription would have worked well in the past, and that this would be the reason for continuing it.

14. A: The word *rises* makes the sentence grammatically correct. At the heart of this question is the distinction between *rise* and *raise*, which can be summed up in one sentence: To *raise* is to cause to *rise*. This probably requires a little explanation. *Raise* is generally a transitive verb, meaning that it has to be done to something. In other words, it needs an object. One *raises* a window or *raises* a question, but a window or question does not *raise* itself. *Rise*, on the other hand, is typically used as an intransitive verb. This means that it does not take an object. I *rise* from sleep; I do not *rise myself* from sleep. In the sentence for question 14, the blood pressure is doing the action described by the verb, and there is no object. For this reason, *rises* is correct.

15. C: The word *despite* completes the sentence correctly. *Despite* is a preposition meaning "notwithstanding" or "in spite of." A preposition is a word that indicates relationship. *At*, *by*, *with*, and *before* are all prepositions. All of the answer choices for question 15 include prepositions. So in order to answer the question, you need to determine which relationship the author is most likely trying to express. The first clause indicates that the two professionals had similar training, and the second clause that indicates they drew different conclusions. It would not make sense for them to draw different conclusions *because of* their similar training; one would expect both professionals to approach a question in the same way. Answer choices B and D create an incoherent statement when they are substituted into the sentence. The answer must therefore be C.

16. D: The word *is* makes the sentence grammatically correct. In order to answer this question correctly, you need to be able to identify the subject. Although it may seem as if the subject is *the two European capitals*, this is actually a clause related to the subject *each*. *Each* is a singular pronoun, in which two or more things are being considered individually. In this case, each of these things is an "it," so the appropriate verb form will be the third-person singular present indicative *is*.

17. B: The word *further* is not used correctly in the context of this sentence. Here, the word *farther* would be more appropriate. The distinction between *further* and *farther* is likely to appear in at least one question on the HESI exam. For the purposes of the examination, you just need to know that *farther* can be used to describe physical distance, while *further* cannot. In this sentence, the speaker is describing a distance to be walked, which is a physical distance. For this reason, the word *further* is incorrect.

18. B: The word *sat* is used incorrectly in this sentence. The word *set* would be a good substitution for *sat*. The distinction between *sit* and *set* is likely to appear at least once during the HESI exam. *Sit* is an intransitive verb that does not need an object. One does not *sit* something else, one just *sits*. *Set*, meanwhile, is a transitive verb that requires an object. One *sets* an alarm clock or a table, one does not just *set*. In the sentence on question 18, the little boy is placing something, namely the red block. A transitive verb is required, therefore. For this reason, the past tense of *set* (also *set*) is correct, while the past tense of *sit* (*sat*) is not.

19. B: The phrase *to divulge* makes the sentence grammatically correct. *To divulge* is the infinitive form of a verb meaning to "reveal or disclose information." The verb can stay in the present tense because the speaker is describing what Laura knew at a particular time in the past. In other words, the author has already established the past tense with the word *knew*. It would also be appropriate to fill this blank with the word *divulging*. However, this is not one of the answer choices.

20. C: The word *closely* makes the sentence grammatically correct. Remember that an adjective is a word that describes a noun, while an adverb describes an adjective, a verb, or another adverb. In this sentence, you are looking for the right word to describe how the attendant *looked*. This means that you are looking for an adverb. Most of the time, adverbs end in *-ly*. On question 20, answer choices C and D both have this ending. Answer choice D, however, does not really make sense when substituted into the sentence.

21. B: The word *illusion* is used incorrectly in this sentence. Instead, the author should have used the word *allusion*. An illusion is a false or deceptive image. For example, a magician pulling a rabbit out a hat is a famous illusion. The magician does not actually produce the rabbit out of thin air, but is able to create the image of having done so. An *allusion*, on the other hand, is an indirect reference. If the doctor had said something like, "in light of your past issues," and Henry knew that the doctor meant his depression, then the doctor would have made an allusion.

22. B: The word *should* correctly completes the sentence. All of the answer choices are auxiliary verbs, which are verbs that accompany other verbs and add some element of tone or mood. In order to determine the appropriate auxiliary verb for this sentence, you need to take a close look at the context. The *if* that initiates the sentence suggests that the author is making a conditional statement. In other words, in order to join the club, a condition must be met: Namely, the coach must be contacted by Thursday. For this reason, *should* is the appropriate auxiliary verb. When should is placed before a verb, it adds a note of obligation or recommendation. For instance, saying "you should brush your teeth" is like saying "brushing your teeth is a healthful act that you ought to do."

23. B: The word *set* makes the sentence grammatically correct. This questions centers on the distinction between *set* and *sit*. *Set* is transitive and needs to have an object. This means that it has to be done to something (there are a few exceptions, like *the sun sets*). The past tense and past participle of *set* are both *set*. *Sit*, meanwhile, is intransitive and takes no object. You don't sit something; you just sit. The past tense and past participle of *sit* is *sat*. In this case, the blank must be filled by a transitive verb, because the verb is acting on something else: the law practice. For this reason, *set* is the correct answer.

24. A: The phrase *more efficient* makes the sentence grammatically correct. Here, the author is attempting to describe a comparison between two things: the coal furnace and the woodstove. The comparative form of an adjective usually ends with *-er*: *taller, wiser, cleaner*, for example. In some cases, however, the word *more* is placed in front of the unchanged adjective. As a general rule, multisyllabic words are more likely to use the *more* construction than the *-er* construction. That is the case with *efficient*. Unfortunately, there is no easy rule for memorizing the comparative forms of common English adjectives. Reading is one way to develop a good eye for proper usage.

25. C: The word *has* is used incorrectly in this sentence. The auxiliary verb *have* would be a correct substitution for *has*. *Have* and *has* are auxiliary verbs that, along with *developed*, form a past participle. A past participle is used for action that took place in the past and is now complete. The subject of the sentence is soccer players, which means the verb has to be in the third-person plural. *Has*, however, is the third-person singular. *Have* is in the third-person plural and would therefore be a better choice.

26. A: The word *him* makes the sentence grammatically correct. In this sentence, the blank needs to be filled by a direct object, because you are looking for the person, place, or thing to which the action of the

verb is being done. Here, we are looking to identify the person who was asked. For that reason, we need the objective case of *he*, which is *him*. The objective case of *she* is *her*. There will probably be several questions in the grammar section of the HESI exam that require you to differentiate between a pronoun used as a subject and a pronoun used as an object.

27. B: The word *with* makes the sentence grammatically correct. *With* is a preposition that can mean a number of different things. Perhaps the most common meaning of *with* is "in the company of." In this sentence, however, a more accurate meaning is "in regard to." The word *among* is not appropriate here, because progress is not something one could physically be in the middle of. That is, *progress* is not a group of individual things. The word *regards* is not grammatically appropriate for this sentence, although the sentence could be correctly completed with the phrase *with regard to*. Finally, the word *besides* is incorrect because it would not make sense for Felix to not be pleased with his own progress.

28. C: The word *hungrily* makes the sentence grammatically correct. In order to answer this question, you must know the difference between an adjective and an adverb. An adjective modifies a noun. For instance, in the phrase *the delicious meatball*, *delicious* is an adjective. An adverb, on the other hand, modifies an adjective, a verb, or another adverb. In the phrase *walking quickly away*, *quickly* is an adverb. In the sentence for this question, it seems clear that the answer must modify the verb *eyed*. After all, it would not make much sense for the cheesecake to be hungry. This means that an adverb is required. The adverbial form of *hungry* is *hungrily*.

29. C: The word *recipe* is not used correctly in the context of this sentence. The author of this sentence has apparently confused the word *recipe* and *receipt*. A *recipe* is a list of instructions for making something, usually a food or beverage. You might have a recipe for chocolate chip cookies, for instance. A *receipt*, on the other hand, is a printed acknowledgement of having received a certain amount of money and goods. The slip of paper you are handed after paying for something in a store is a receipt. The HESI exam will most likely contain a few questions that require you to identify mixed-up word choices.

30. B: The word *good* properly completes this sentence. This question centers on the distinction between good and well, and, more generally, between adjectives and adverbs. An adjective is used to describe a noun or a pronoun. In the phrase *the red bicycle*, for example, *red* is an adjective describing *bicycle*. An adverb, on the other hand, describes a verb, an adjective, or another adverb. Words that end in *-ly* are usually adverbs, describing the way something is done. As an example, in the phrase *running steadily*, *steadily* is an adverb. To succeed on the HESI exam, you need to know that *good* is an adjective and *well* is an adverb. In question 30, you are looking for a word that describes how Sharon felt, not one that describes her act of feeling. For this reason, you should select the adjective *good*.

31. D: The word *lying* is used incorrectly in this sentence. It would be correct to use the verb *laying* instead. The distinction between *laying* and *lying* is tricky. *Laying* is typically used as a transitive verb, meaning that it is done to something. One lays bricks or lays carpet, for instance. Lie, on the other hand, is an intransitive verb: It is not done to something; it is just done. You *lie* on the floor, for instance. The definition of *lay* is to place; to *lie* is to take a horizontal position. In this sentence, the subject (Brendan) is laying something (bricks), so it is incorrect to use the verb *lying*.

32. A: The word *who* makes the sentence grammatically correct. In this sentence, *who* is being used as a relative pronoun: that is, a pronoun introducing a clause that describes a noun already mentioned. The noun being referred to, known as the antecedent, is *children*. Because children are people with a personality and identity, the pronoun *who* is used rather than *which*. *Which* is used as a relative pronoun when the antecedent is an inanimate object, such as a box or a house.

33. C: The word *struck* makes the sentence grammatically correct. *Struck* is the past tense and past participle of *strike*, meaning "to hit" or "to beat." *Striked* is not a word. In this case, however, the author is using the common expression "struck a bargain." This expression is frequently used to describe deal making or the end of negotiations. These kinds of conversational phrases may be especially difficult for students whose native language is not English. If you are unfamiliar with expressions in English, you may want to pick up a glossary of slang or colloquial expressions.

34. A: The phrase *him or her* makes the sentence grammatically correct. In this case, we are looking for a word or words that can serve as the object of the preposition *for*. *She* and *he* are nominative forms, meaning that they can only be used as the subject of a sentence or a clause. *Them* can be the object of a preposition, but it is plural and, therefore, cannot correctly refer to the singular subject *a child*. (Incidentally, the use of *they* and *them* to refer to a singular subject is one of the most common grammatical errors, and will almost certainly appear in one or more questions on the HESI exam.) For a similar reason, you cannot use *it* to refer to *a child*. The correct answer, then, is *him or her*.

35. A: The word *swam* makes the sentence grammatically correct. *Swam* is the past tense of the verb *swim*. The context of this sentence makes clear that the action took place in the past; the author uses the past tense verb *was* and describes an action that has already been completed. *Swimmed* is an incorrect verb form. *Swum* is the past participle of *swim*; it would be appropriate if the sentence read *he had swum* or *he has swum*. The absence of these auxiliary verbs means that the simple past tense is appropriate here.

36. C: The phrase *she and I* makes the sentence grammatically correct. The blank needs to be filled by the subject of the sentence. The subject of a sentence or clause is the person, place, or thing that performs the verb. There are a couple of ways to determine that this sentence needs a subject. To begin with, the blank is at the beginning of the sentence, where the subject most often is found. Also, when you read the sentence, you will notice that it is unclear who went to the movies. Because you are looking for the subject, you need the nominative pronouns *she and I*.

37. C: The word *set* makes the sentence grammatically correct. This question requires knowledge of the distinction between *set* and *sit*. *Set* is a transitive verb meaning "to place in a particular position." Transitive verbs have to be done *to* something. *Sit*, meanwhile, is an intransitive verb meaning "to assume a seated posture." In this case, Brian is performing the action of the verb on something in particular: the alarm clock. For this reason, the verb *set* is appropriate.

38. B: The word *shaked* is incorrect in this sentence. In fact, *shaked* is not a word at all. The past tense of *shake* is *shook*. This is similar to the word *take*, which has as its past tense *took* rather than *taked*. There is no real reason for this, making it yet another usage pattern in English that does not conform to any strict rules. After all, the past tense of *wake* is *waked* rather than *wook*. There is no easy way to know all of these rules and exceptions, but a good way to acquire a sense of standard English usage is to become widely read and use a dictionary.

39. B: The word *whichever* makes the sentence grammatically correct. In this sentence, *whichever* is being used as an adjective modifying *way*. The presence of this adjective indicates that Ted was looking in any number of different ways. *Moreover* is an adverb meaning "in addition" or "besides." *Whomever* is the form of whoever used as a direct object, indirect object, or object of a preposition. *Whether* is a conjunction that suggests alternatives or sets of two choices.

40. C: The word *lain* properly completes the sentence. On this question, the presence of the word *had* is the biggest clue to the right answer. *Had* indicates that the verb phrase is being used as a past participle. A past participle is the verb form used to describe action that took place in the past and has been completed. In other words, the treasure started lying there a long time ago, and its position was fully established in

- 136 -

the past. Remember that *lain* is the past participle of *lie*, and *laid* is the past participle of *lay*. The verb here is clearly intransitive (that is, it does not act on something else, it just does something), so the correct form is *lain*.

41. B: The word *fewer* makes the sentence grammatically correct. The distinction between fewer and less will most likely appear on your HESI exam. In general, *fewer* is used for things that can be counted and *less* is used for things that cannot be counted. So, for instance, one would say "fewer attendees at this year's conference" and "less confidence in the economy." In this sentence, the adjective is modifying *patients*, who of course can be counted quite easily. So, the correct answer is *fewer*.

42. B: The word *after* makes the sentence grammatically correct. *After* is a conjunction meaning "behind in place or position." A conjunction is a part of speech that connects different words, phrase, and ideas. *And*, *but*, and *because* are all conjunctions. In order to find the appropriate word to complete the sentence in question 42, you need to take a close look at the context. The sentence indicates that Kim realized she had forgotten her list of questions at some time relating to the interview. In other words, it seems clear that the blank must be completed with some word relating to time. Kim either made this realization before, during, or after the interview. Since *after* is one of the answer choices, it must be the correct answer.

43. D: The word *one* is used incorrectly in this sentence. Here, *one* is being used as a pronoun: a stand-in for some other noun. The problem is that it is unclear to what it is referring. The only possible reference for *one* is video store, and it does not make sense to say that "we should rent a video store." Most of the time, we would read this sentence and just assume that the author meant that we should rent a video. However, on the HESI exam, you must be alert for unclear wording.

44. A: The word *who* makes this sentence correct. *Who* is an interrogative pronoun that can be either singular or plural. A pronoun is a word that stands in for another noun. In this case, the pronoun is used so that the author can inquire about the noun to which the pronoun is referring. Once the question is answered, the names of the best eye doctors could be substituted for *who* to make a complete sentence. In any case, *who* is appropriate because the pronoun is referring to people who have both personality and identity; if they were objects, it would be appropriate to use *which* or *what*. *Whom* is a pronoun in the objective cases and is therefore not appropriate for this sentence.

45. B: The word *spent* makes this sentence grammatically correct. The sentence is clearly describing action that took place in the past, because the introductory clause begins with the word *while*. It cannot be determined whether this action is ongoing or has been completed. The past tense of the verb *spend* is *spent*. Unfortunately, there is no rule to guide this past tense; as a matter of fact, the past tense of the verb *mend* is *mended*, which might lead you to believe that *spended* is correct. Reading a variety of materials is the best way to develop an ear for proper usage.

46. A: The word *amount* correctly completes this sentence. This question centers on the distinction between *amount* and *number*. An *amount* is a quantity that cannot be counted, while a *number* is a quantity that can be counted. There is no way to count pain, so *amount* is a better word choice than *number*. *Frequency* is rate of occurrence, or how often something happens. If a doctor asks how often a patient gets a migraine, for instance, she is asking about the *frequency* of the headaches. *Amplitude* is the specific breadth or width. Amplitude is mainly used to describe waves; the difference in height between the top of a wave (crest) and the bottom (trough) is the amplitude.

47. C: The word *their* is used incorrectly in this sentence. The problem is that *whoever* as it is used here is a singular subject, while *their* is a plural possessive pronoun. *Whoever* can be either singular or plural, depending on how it is used. In this case, however, because the author is describing a letter writer who

forgot to sign the letter, it seems clear that *whoever* is meant as a singular. For this reason, the author should use *his or her* instead of *their*.

48. C: The word *too* makes the sentence grammatically correct. Clearly, the author is trying to express that the child's fever was excessively high. Of the four answer choices, three convey this idea. Only answer choice A (the preposition *to*) can be immediately eliminated. The best way to find the final answer is to substitute each of the answer choices into the sentence and read the result. Answer choice B requires the addition of the word *too* to make any sense. Answer choice C, then, must be the correct answer.

49. B: The word *presents* makes the sentence grammatically correct. The author is referring to the symptoms that will be displayed when a patient has a particular condition: that is, the presentation of the condition. Because the subject of the sentence (*condition*) is singular, it is proper to use the verb form ending in an *s*. For this reason, you should select answer choice B rather than answer choice C. *Presence* is the quality of being there. When a teacher is calling roll and a student responds to his name by saying "present," he is using a form of this word to indicate that he is there. Of course, *present* can also mean a gift. *Prescience*, on the other hand, is foreknowledge, or knowledge ahead of time. You can exercise prescience by learning the content of the HESI exam and practicing with this study guide.

50. B: The preposition *among* is not used correctly in the context of the sentence. In this case, the word *between* would be more appropriate. *Among* and *between* both mean "in the midst of some other things." However, *between* is used when there are only two other things, and *among* is used when there are more than two. For example, it would be correct to say "between first and second base" or "among several friends." In this sentence, the preposition *among* is inappropriate for describing placement amid "two treatment protocols."

Mathematics Questions

1. 474 + 2038 =
   a. 2512
   b. 2412
   c. 2521
   d. 2502

2. 32,788 + 1693 =
   a. 33,481
   b. 32,383
   c. 34,481
   d. 36,481

3. 3703 − 1849 =
   a. 1954
   b. 1854
   c. 1974
   d. 1794

4. 4790 − 2974 =
   a. 1816
   b. 1917
   c. 2109
   d. 1779

5. 229 × 738 =
    a. 161,622
    b. 167,670
    c. 169,002
    d. 171,451

6. 356 × 808 =
    a. 274,892
    b. 278,210
    c. 283,788
    d. 287,648

7. Round to the nearest whole number: 435 ÷ 7 =
    a. 16
    b. 62
    c. 74
    d. 86

8. Round to the nearest whole number: 4748 ÷ 12 =
    a. 372
    b. 384
    c. 396
    d. 412

9. Report all decimal places: 3.7 + 7.289 + 4 =
    a. 14.989
    b. 5.226
    c. 15.0
    d. 15.07

10. 4.934 + 7.1 + 9.08 =
    a. 21.114
    b. 21.042
    c. 20.214
    d. 59.13

11. 27 – 3.54 =
    a. 24.56
    b. 23.46
    c. 33.3
    d. 24.54

12. 28.19 – 9 =
    a. 28.1
    b. 18.19
    c. 27.29
    d. 19.19

13. Karen goes to the grocery store with $40. She buys a carton of milk for $1.85, a loaf of bread for $3.20, and a bunch of bananas for $3.05. How much money does she have left?
   a. $30.95
   b. $31.90
   c. $32.10
   d. $34.95

14. Round your answer to the tenths place: $0.088 \times 277.9 =$
   a. 21.90
   b. 2.5
   c. 24.5
   d. 24.46

15. Round your answer to the hundredths place: $28 \div 0.6 =$
   a. 46.67
   b. 0.021
   c. 17.50
   d. 16.8

16. Roger's car gets an average of 25 miles per gallon. If his gas tank holds 16 gallons, about how far can he drive on a full tank?
   a. 41 miles
   b. 100 miles
   c. 320 miles
   d. 400 miles

17. Express the answer in simplest form: $\dfrac{3}{8} + \dfrac{2}{8} =$

   a. $\dfrac{1}{8}$

   b. $\dfrac{1}{2}$

   c. $\dfrac{5}{8}$

   d. $\dfrac{5}{16}$

18. Express the answer in simplest form: $\dfrac{2}{3} + \dfrac{2}{7} =$

   a. $\dfrac{20}{21}$

   b. $\dfrac{4}{10}$

   c. $\dfrac{4}{21}$

   d. $\dfrac{2}{5}$

19. Present the sum as a mixed number in simplest form: $1\frac{1}{2} + \frac{12}{9} =$

a. $2\frac{3}{5}$

b. $1\frac{3}{4}$

c. $3\frac{1}{3}$

d. $2\frac{5}{6}$

20. Aaron worked $2\frac{1}{2}$ hours on Monday, $3\frac{3}{4}$ hours on Tuesday, and $7\frac{2}{3}$ hours on Thursday. How many hours did he work in all?

a. $10\frac{5}{6}$

b. $12\frac{1}{2}$

c. $13\frac{1}{4}$

d. $13\frac{11}{12}$

21. Express the answer in simplest form: $\frac{23}{24} - \frac{11}{24} =$

a. $\frac{11}{23}$

b. $\frac{1}{2}$

c. $\frac{2}{3}$

d. $\frac{12}{24}$

22. Express the answer in simplest form: $3\frac{4}{7} - 2\frac{3}{14} =$

a. $2\frac{3}{14}$

b. $1\frac{1}{14}$

c. $1\frac{5}{14}$

d. $2\frac{3}{7}$

23. Express the answer in simplest form: Dean has brown, white, and black socks. One-third of his socks are white; one-sixth of his socks are black. How many of his socks are brown?

a. $\frac{1}{3}$

b. $\frac{2}{6}$

c. $\frac{1}{2}$

d. $\frac{3}{4}$

24. Express the answer in simplest form: A recipe calls for $1\frac{1}{2}$ cups sugar, $3\frac{2}{3}$ cups flour, and $\frac{2}{3}$ cup milk. If you want to double the recipe, what will be the total amount of cups of ingredients required?

a. $11\frac{2}{3}$

b. 8

c. $12\frac{1}{6}$

d. $6\frac{2}{3}$

25. Express your answer as a mixed number in simplest form: $4\frac{1}{3} \times \frac{2}{7} =$

a. $6\frac{1}{3}$

b. $3\frac{7}{10}$

c. $\frac{8}{21}$

d. $1\frac{5}{21}$

26. Express the answer as a mixed number or fraction in simplest form: $2\frac{3}{9} \times \frac{1}{3} =$

    a. $\frac{7}{8}$

    b. $2\frac{3}{7}$

    c. $\frac{12}{27}$

    d. $\frac{7}{9}$

27. Express the answer as a mixed number or fraction in simplest form: $\frac{5}{8} \div \frac{1}{5} =$

    a. $\frac{1}{8}$

    b. $2\frac{3}{4}$

    c. $3\frac{1}{3}$

    d. $3\frac{1}{8}$

28. Express the answer as a mixed number or fraction in simplest form: $\frac{2}{7} \div \frac{1}{6} =$

    a. $\frac{1}{21}$

    b. $2\frac{1}{12}$

    c. $1\frac{3}{4}$

    d. $1\frac{5}{7}$

29. Round to the nearest whole number: Bill got $\frac{7}{9}$ of the answers right on his chemistry test. On a scale of 1 to 100, what numerical grade would he receive?

    a. 77
    b. 78
    c. 79
    d. 80

30. Round to the hundredths place. Change the fraction to a decimal: $\frac{7}{8}$ =

   a. 0.88
   b. 0.92
   c. 0.84
   d. 0.78

31. Round to the hundredths place. Change the fraction to a decimal: $4\frac{3}{7}$ =

   a. 4.37
   b. 4.43
   c. 4.56
   d. 4.78

32. Change the decimal to the simplest equivalent proper fraction: 3.78 =

   a. $3\frac{3}{4}$

   b. $3\frac{7}{8}$

   c. $3\frac{39}{50}$

   d. $3\frac{78}{100}$

33. Change the decimal to the simplest equivalent proper fraction: 0.07 =

   a. $\frac{7}{10}$

   b. $\frac{0.07}{10}$

   c. $\frac{7}{100}$

   d. $\frac{70}{100}$

34. Change the decimal to the simplest equivalent proper fraction: 2.80 =

   a. $\frac{2.8}{10}$

   b. $2\frac{8}{10}$

   c. $\frac{0.28}{1}$

   d. $2\frac{4}{5}$

35. Change the fraction to the simplest possible ratio: $\dfrac{8}{14}$

    a. 2:3
    b. 4:7
    c. 4:6
    d. 3:5

36. Two-thirds of the students in Mr. Garcia's class are boys. If there are 27 students in the class, how many of them are girls?

    a. 1
    b. 9
    c. 12
    d. 20

37. Solve for x:
3:2 :: 24:x
    a. 16
    b. 12
    c. 2
    d. 22

38. Solve for x:
7:42 :: 4:x
    a. 12
    b. 48
    c. 24
    d. 16

39. Change the decimal to a percent: 0.64 =
    a. 0.64%
    b. 64%
    c. 6.4%
    d. 0.064%

40. Change the decimal to a percent: 0.000026 =
    a. 0.0026%
    b. 0.026%
    c. 2.6%
    d. 26%

41. Change the percent to a decimal: 38% =
    a. 3.8
    b. 0.038
    c. 38.0
    d. 0.38

42. Change the percent to a decimal: 17.6% =
   a. 17.6
   b. 1.76
   c. 0.176
   d. 0.0176

43. Change the percent to a decimal: 126% =
   a. 126.0
   b. 0.0126
   c. 0.126
   d. 1.26

44. Round to the nearest whole number. Change the fraction to a percent: $\dfrac{2}{9}$ =
   a. 20%
   b. 21%
   c. 22%
   d. 23%

45. Round to the nearest whole number. Change the fraction to a percent: $\dfrac{9}{13}$ =
   a. 33%
   b. 69%
   c. 72%
   d. 78%

46. Round to the nearest whole number: What is 17 out of 68, as a percent?
   a. 17%
   b. 25%
   c. 32%
   d. 68%

47. Round to the nearest percentage point: Gerald made 13 out of the 22 shots he took in the basketball game. What was his shooting percentage?
   a. 13%
   b. 22%
   c. 59%
   d. 67%

48. Round to the nearest whole number: What is 18% of 600?
   a. 108
   b. 76
   c. 254
   d. 176

49. Round to the tenths place: What is 6.4% of 32?
   a. 1.8
   b. 2.1
   c. 2.6
   d. 2.0

50. What is the numerical value of the Roman number XVII?
    a. 22
    b. 17
    c. 48
    d. 57

Mathematics Answer Key and Explanations

1. A: The answer is 2512. To solve this problem, you must know how to add numbers with multiple digits. It may be easier for you to complete this problem if you align the numbers vertically. The crucial thing when setting up the vertical problem is to make sure that the place values are lined up correctly. In this problem, the larger number (2038) should be placed on top, such that the 8 is over the 4, the 3 is over the 7, and so on. Then add the place value farthest to the right. In this case, the 4 and the 8 that we find in the ones place have a sum of 12; the 2 is placed in the final sum, and the 1 is carried over to the next place value to the left, the tens. The tens place is the next to be added: 3 plus 7 equal 10, with the addition of the carried 1 making 11. Again, the first 1 is carried over to the next place value. The problem proceeds on in this vein.

2. C: The answer is 34,481. This problem requires you to understand addition of multiple-digit numbers. As in the first problem, the most important step is properly aligning the two addends in vertical formation, such that the final 8 in 32,788 is above the final 3 in 1693. Again, as in the first problem, you will be required to carry numbers over. It is a good idea to practice these addition problems and pay special attention to carrying over, since errors in this area can produce answers that look correct. The administrators of the HESI exam will sometimes try to take advantage of these common errors by making a couple of the wrong answers the results one would get by failing to carry over a digit.

3. B: The answer is 1854. To solve this problem, you must know how to subtract one multiple-digit number from another. As with the above addition problems, the most important step in this kind of problem is to set up the proper vertical alignment. In subtraction problems, the larger number must always be on top, and there can be only two terms in all (an addition problem can have an infinite number of terms). In this problem, the ones places should be aligned such that the 3 in 3703 is above the 9 in 1849. This problem also requires you to understand what to do when you have a larger value on the bottom of a subtraction problem. In this case, the 3 on the top of the ones place is smaller than the 9 beneath it, so it must borrow 1 from the number to its left. Unfortunately, there is a 0 to the left of the three, so we must extract a 1 from the next place over again. The 7 in 3703 becomes a 6, the 0 becomes a 10 only to have 1 taken away, leaving it as a 9. The 3 in the ones place becomes 13, from which we can now subtract the 9.

4. A: The answer is 1816. This problem requires you to understand subtraction with multiple-digit numbers. As in problem 3, the most important step is to align the problem vertically such that the 0 in 4790 is above the 4 in 2974. Again as in problem 3, you will have to borrow from the place value to the left when the number on the bottom is bigger than the number on top. Be sure to practice this kind of problem with special attention to borrowing from adjacent place values. The HESI exam will often include a few wrong answers that you could mistakenly derive by simply forgetting how to borrow.

5. C: The answer is 169,002. To solve this problem, you must know how to multiply numbers with several digits. These problems often intimidate students because they produce such large numbers, but they are actually quite simple. As with the above addition and subtraction problems, the crucial first step is to align the terms vertically such that the 8 in 738 is above the 9 in 229. In multiplication, it is a good idea to

put the larger number on top, although it is only essential to do so when one of the terms has more place values than the other. In a multiple-digit multiplication problem, every digit gets multiplied by every other digit: First the 9 in 229 is multiplied by the three digits in 738, moving from right to left. Only the digit in the ones place is brought down; the digit in the tens place is placed above the digit to the immediate left and added to the product of the next multiplication. In this problem, then, the 9 and 8 produce 72: The 2 is placed below, and the 7 is placed above the 3 in 738. Then the 9 and the 3 are multiplied and produce 27, to which the 7 is added, making 24. The 4 comes down, the 2 goes above the first 2 in 229, and the process continues. The product of 9 multiplied by 738 is placed below and is added to the products of 2 and 738 and 2 and 738, respectively. For each successive product, the first digit goes one place value to the left. So, in other words, 0 is placed under the 2. These three products are added together to calculate the final product of 738 and 229.

6. D: The answer is 287,648. This problem requires you to understand multiplication of numbers with several digits. The difficulties you may face with this problem are identical to those of problem 5. Be sure set up your vertical alignment properly, such that the 8 in 808 is above the 6 in 356. Multiply the 6 in 356 by 8, 0, and 8, proceeding from right to left. Then multiply the 5 in 356 by 8, 0, and 8; finally, multiply the 3 in 356 by 8. For each successive product, add one zero at the extreme right of the product. Add the three products together to find your final answer.

7. B: The answer is 62. To solve this problem, you must know how to divide a multiple-digit number by a single-digit number. To begin with, set up the problem as $7\overline{)435}$. Then determine the number of times that 7 will go into 43 (one way to do this is to multiply 7 by various numbers until you find a product that is either 43 exactly or no more than 6 fewer than 43). In this case, you will find that 7 goes into 43 six times. Place the 6 above the 3 in 435 and multiply the 6 by 7. The product, 42, should be subtracted from 43, leaving a difference of 1. Since 7 cannot go into 1, bring down the 5 to create 15. The 7 will go into 15 twice, so place a 2 to the right of the 6 on top of the problem. At this point, you should recognize that only answer choice B can be correct. If you proceed further, however, you will find that 435 must become 435.0 so that the 0 can be brought down to make a large enough number to be divided by 7. Once a decimal point is introduced to the dividend, a decimal point must be placed directly above it in the quotient. If you continue working this problem, you will end up with an answer of 62.14 … Note that the instructions tell you only to round to the nearest whole number. Once you have solved to the tenths place, there is no need to continue.

8. C: The answer is 396. To solve this problem, you must understand division involving multiple-digit numbers. To begin with, set up the problem as $12\overline{)4,748}$. Then solve the problem according to the procedure you followed in problem 7. Since you are asked to round to the nearest whole number, you must solve this problem to the tenths place. If your calculations are correct, you will have a 6 in the tenths place, meaning that the answer should be rounded up from 395 to 396.

9. A: The answer is 14.989. To solve this problem, you must know how to add a series of numbers when some of the numbers include decimals. As with addition problems 1 and 2, the most important first step is to set up the proper vertical alignment. This step is even more important when working with decimals. Be sure that all of the decimal points are in alignment; in other words, the 7 in 3.7 should be above the 2 in 7.289. Since the final term, 4, is a whole number, we assume a 0 in the tenths place. Similarly, you may assume zeros in the hundredths and thousandths places, if you prefer to have a digit in every relevant place. Then beginning at the rightmost place value (in this case, the thousandths), add the terms together as you would with whole numbers. The decimal point of the sum should be aligned with the decimal points of the terms.

10. A: The answer is 21.114. This problem requires you to understand addition involving a series of numbers, some of which include decimals. This problem is solved in the same manner as problem 9. Be sure to align the terms correctly, such that the 9 in 4.934 is above the 1 in 7.1 and the 0 in 9.08. Assume zeros for the hundredths and thousandths place of 7.1 and for the thousandths place of 9.08. The usual rules for carrying in addition still apply when working with decimals.

11. B: The answer is 23.46. To solve this problem, you must know how to subtract a number with a decimal from a whole number. At first glance, this problem seems complex, but it is actually quite simple once you set it up in a vertical form. Remember that the decimal point must remain aligned and that a decimal point can be assumed after the 7 in 27. In order to solve this problem, you should assume zeros for the tenths and hundredths places of 27. The problem is solved as 27.00 – 3.54. Obviously, in order to solve this problem you will have to borrow from the 7 in 27.00. The normal rules for borrowing in subtraction still apply when working with decimals. Be sure to keep the decimal point of the difference aligned with the decimal points of the terms.

12. D: The answer is 19.19. This problem requires you to understand subtraction of a whole number from a number with a decimal. This problem is somewhat similar to problem 11, although here the decimal is on the top in your vertical alignment. Assume zeros for the tenths and hundredths place of the bottom term, creating the problem 28.19 – 9.00. Be sure to keep your decimal point in the same position in the difference as in the terms. HESI exam administrators often try to fool test-takers by including some possible answers that have the correct digits, but in which the decimal point is misplaced.

13. B: The answer is $31.90. To solve this problem, you must know how to solve word problems involving decimal subtraction. In this scenario, Karen starts out with a certain amount of money and spends some of it on groceries. To calculate how much money she has left, simply subtract the money spent from the original figure: 40 – 1.85 – 3.20 – 3.05. There is no reason to include the dollar sign in your calculations, so long as you remember that it exists. You cannot subtract the costs of these items at the same time, so you must either subtract them one by one or add them up and subtract the sum from 40. Either way will generate the right answer.

14. C: The answer is 24.5. This problem requires you to understand multiplication including numbers with decimals. In some ways, multiplying decimals is easier than adding or subtracting them. This is because the decimal points can be ignored until the very end of the process. Simply set this problem up such that the longer term, 277.9, is on top (this term is considered longer because the initial 0 in 0.088 performs no function). Then multiply according to the usual system: Multiply the rightmost 8 by 9, 7, 7, and 2, and then do the same for the next 8. Add the two products together. Finally, count up the number of decimal places to the right of the decimal point in both terms. In this problem, there are four: 0.<u>088</u> and 277.<u>9</u>. This means that there should be four places to the right of the decimal point in the product. Once the product is found, you must round it to the tenths place. This is done by assessing the digit in the place to the right of the tenths place (that is, the hundredths place). If that digit is lower than 5, round down; if it is 5 or greater, round up. In this case, there is a 5 in the hundredths place, so the 4 in the tenths place becomes a 5.

15. A: The answer is 46.67. To solve this problem, you must know how to divide a whole number by a decimal. To begin with, set the problem up in the form $0.6\overline{)28}$. You cannot perform division when the divisor is less than one, however, so shift the decimal point one place to the right. For every action in the divisor, an identical action must be taken in the dividend: Shift the decimal point (which can be assumed after the 8 in 28) in the dividend as well. The problem is now $6\overline{)280}$. This problem can now be solved just like problems 7 and 8. Remember to round your answer to the hundredths place for this problem

(this means you will need to solve to the thousandths place). With a knowledge of place value, you can immediately eliminate answer choices B and D, since they are solved to the nearest thousandth and tenth place, respectively.

16. D: The answer is 400 miles. This problem requires you to understand word problems involving mileage rates and multiplication. The problem states that the car gets an average 25 miles per gallon; in other words, every gallon of fuel powers the car for approximately 25 miles. If the car holds 16 gallons of gas, then, and each of these gallons provides 25 miles of travel, you can set up the following equation: 25 miles/gallon × 16 gallons = 400 miles. Since the first term has gallons in the denominator and the second term has gallons in what would be the numerator (if it were expressed as 16 gallons/1), these units cancel each other out and leave only miles.

17. C: The answer is $\frac{5}{8}$. To solve this problem, you must know how to add fractions with like denominators. This kind of operation is actually quite simple. The denominator of the sum remains the same; the calculation is performed by adding the numerators. On problems like this, HESI exam administrators will probably try to fool you by including one possible answer in which the denominators have been added; in this problem, for instance, you would end up with answer choice D if you added both numerator and denominator. Do not assume that you have answered the question correctly because your calculations match one of the answer choices. Always check your work.

18. A: The answer is $\frac{20}{21}$. This problem requires you to understand addition of fractions with unlike denominators. The denominator is the bottom term in a fraction; the top term is called the numerator. In order to perform addition with a fraction, all of the terms must have the same denominator. In order to derive the lowest common denominator in this problem, you must list the multiples for 3 and 7 until you find one that both have in common. In increasing order, multiples of 3 are 3, 6, 9, 12, 15, 18, and 21; multiples of 7 are 7, 14, and 21. The lowest common multiple is 21. This is also the lowest common denominator for the two fractions. To convert each term into a fraction with this common denominator, you must multiply both numerator and denominator by the same number. To make the denominator of $\frac{2}{3}$ into 21, you must multiply by 7; therefore, you must also multiply the numerator, 2, by 7. The new fraction is $\frac{14}{21}$. For the second term, you must multiply numerator and denominator by 3: $\frac{2}{7} \times \frac{3}{3} = \frac{6}{21}$. The new addition problem is $\frac{14}{21} + \frac{6}{21}$. Remember that when adding fractions, only the numerators are combined.

19. D: The answer is $2\frac{5}{6}$. To solve this problem, you must know how to add mixed numbers and improper fractions. To begin with, convert the mixed number (a mixed number includes a whole number and a fraction) into an improper fraction (a fraction in which the numerator is larger than the denominator). This is done by multiplying the whole number by the denominator and adding the product to the numerator: 1 × 2 + 1 = 3. The problem is now $\frac{3}{2} + \frac{12}{9}$. Then find the lowest common denominator by listing some multiples of 2 and 9. The lowest common multiple is 18, so you must convert both terms: $\frac{3}{2} \times \frac{9}{9} = \frac{27}{18}$, and $\frac{12}{9} \times \frac{2}{2} = \frac{24}{18}$. The problem is now $\frac{27}{18} + \frac{24}{18} = \frac{51}{18}$. This fraction is converted into a mixed

- 150 -

number by dividing the numerator by the denominator: $\frac{51}{18} = 2\frac{15}{18}$, which can be simplified to $2\frac{5}{6}$ by dividing both numerator and denominator by 3.

20. D: The answer is $13\frac{11}{12}$. This problem requires you to understand addition involving mixed numbers. The calculation required by this problem is straightforward: In order to derive the number of hours worked by Aaron, add up the three mixed numbers. To make this possible, you will need to find the lowest common multiple of 2, 4, and 3, so that you can establish a common denominator. The lowest common denominator for this problem is 12. You can either add up the whole numbers separately from the fractions or convert the mixed numbers into improper fractions and add them in that form. Either way will yield the correct answer.

21. B: The answer is $\frac{1}{2}$. To solve this problem, you must understand subtraction involving fractions with like denominators. As with addition involving fractions with like denominators, you should only subtract the numerators. So, this problem is solved $\frac{23}{24} - \frac{11}{24} = \frac{12}{24}$. This answer can be simplified by dividing by the greatest common factor (a factor is any number that can be divided into the given number equally). The factors of 12 are 1, 2, 3, 4, 6, and 12. The factors of 24 are 1, 2, 3, 4, 6, 8, 12, and 24. The greatest common factor of 12 and 24, then, is 12. Divide both numerator and denominator by 12 to derive the answer in simplest form: $(\frac{12}{12})/(\frac{24}{12}) = \frac{1}{2}$.

22. C: The answer is $1\frac{5}{14}$. This problem requires you to understand subtraction with mixed numbers. In order to perform this problem, you must convert these mixed numbers into improper fractions with the same denominator. Remember that mixed numbers are converted into improper fractions by multiplying the denominator by the whole number and adding the product to the numerator: $3\frac{4}{7}$ becomes $\frac{25}{7}$, and

$2\frac{3}{14}$ becomes $\frac{31}{14}$. Next, find the lowest common denominator by listing multiples of 7 and 14. Since 14 is a multiple of 7, you only have to alter the first term. Multiply both numerator and denominator by 2: $\frac{25}{7} \times \frac{2}{2} = \frac{50}{14}$. The problem is now $\frac{50}{14} - \frac{31}{14} = \frac{19}{14}$. Convert this improper fraction into a mixed number by dividing the numerator by the denominator: $\frac{19}{14} = 1\frac{5}{14}$. The mixed number cannot be simplified further.

23. C: The answer is $\frac{1}{2}$. To solve this problem, you must know how to solve word problems requiring fraction addition and subtraction. You are given the proportions of Dean's socks that are white and black. The best approach to this problem is adding together the two known quantities and subtracting the sum from 1. First you need to find a common denominator for $\frac{1}{3}$ and $\frac{1}{6}$. The lowest common multiple of these two numbers is 6, so convert $\frac{1}{3}$ by multiplying the numerator and denominator by 2. The new equation

will be $\frac{2}{6} + \frac{1}{6} = \frac{3}{6}$. This sum is equivalent to $\frac{1}{2}$, meaning that half of Dean's socks are either white or black. The other half, then, are brown. If you need to perform the calculation, however, it will look like this:

$$\frac{2}{2} - \frac{1}{2} = \frac{1}{2}.$$

24. A: The answer is $11\frac{2}{3}$. This problem requires you to understand word problems involving the addition and multiplication of mixed numbers and improper fractions. To begin with, convert the three mixed numbers to improper fractions by multiplying the whole number by the denominator and adding the product to the numerator. The resulting fractions will be $\frac{3}{2}$ (sugar), $\frac{11}{3}$ (flour), and $\frac{2}{3}$ (milk). Then find the lowest common multiple of 2 and 3 which is 6 and convert the three fractions so that they have this denominator: $\frac{9}{6}$ (sugar), $\frac{22}{6}$ (flour), and $\frac{4}{6}$ (milk). Add these fractions together and multiply the sum by two to double the recipe: $\frac{9}{6} + \frac{22}{6} + \frac{4}{6} = \frac{35}{6} \times 2 = \frac{70}{6}$ Finally, convert this improper fraction to a simple mixed number by dividing numerator by denominator and simplifying the leftover fraction:

$$\frac{70}{6} = 11\frac{4}{6} = 11\frac{2}{3}.$$

25. D: The answer is $1\frac{5}{21}$. To solve this problem, you must know how to multiply mixed numbers and fractions. Unlike fraction addition and subtraction, fraction multiplication does not require a common denominator. However, it is necessary to convert mixed numbers into improper fractions. This is done by multiplying the whole number by the denominator and adding the product to the numerator: in this case, $4 \times 3 + 1 = 13$. So the problem is now $\frac{13}{3} \times \frac{2}{7}$. Fraction multiplication is performed by multiplying numerator by numerator and denominator by denominator: $(13 \times 2)/(3 \times 7) = \frac{26}{21}$. This improper fraction can be converted into a mixed number by dividing numerator by denominator, which gives $1\frac{5}{21}$. Note that since 26 and 21 have no common factors other than 1, the improper fraction cannot be simplified.

26. D: The answer is $\frac{7}{9}$. This problem requires you to understand multiplication of mixed numbers and fractions. The process is the same as for the previous problem: Convert $2\frac{3}{9}$ into the mixed number $\frac{21}{9}$ (if you like, you can simplify this fraction by dividing top and bottom by 3). Then multiply numerator by numerator and denominator by denominator. If you did not simplify the first fraction, you will have a product of $\frac{21}{27}$. This fraction can be simplified by dividing the numerator and denominator by 3: $(21/3)/(27/3) = 7/9$.

27. D: The answer is $3\frac{1}{8}$. To solve this problem, you must know how to divide fractions. The process of dividing fractions is similar to that of multiplying fractions, except that the second term must be inverted. Once this is done, the numerator is multiplied by the numerator, and the denominator is multiplied by the denominator. The inversion of a number is also known as the reciprocal. So, in this problem, solve by multiplying $\frac{5}{8}$ by the reciprocal of $\frac{1}{5}$, which is $\frac{5}{1}$ (finding the reciprocal of a fraction simply means switching the numerator with the denominator). The problem is solved as $(5 \times 5)/(8 \times 1) = \frac{25}{8}$. Convert this improper fraction into a mixed number according to the usual procedure.

28. D: The answer is $1\frac{5}{7}$. This problem requires you to understand how to divide fractions. The procedure is the same as for the previous problem: Invert the second term and change the problem to one of multiplication: $2/7 \times 6/1 = \frac{12}{7}$. Convert this improper fraction into a mixed number according to the usual procedure. The fraction cannot be simplified because 12 and 7 do not share any factors other than 1.

29. B: The answer is 78. To solve this problem, you must know how to convert a fraction into a ratio. In this problem, you are being asked to convert the fraction into a value on a scale from 1 to 100, which is basically like being asked to convert it into a percentage. To do so, divide the numerator by the denominator. The answer will be a repeating seven: $0.7\overline{777}$. Calculate to the thousandth place in order to determine the value. Because the digit in the thousandths place is a 7, you will round up the digit to the left to establish the final answer, 78.

30. A: The answer is 0.88. This problem requires you to understand the conversion of fractions to decimals. The process is fairly simple: Divide the numerator by the denominator. In order to make this possible, you will have to write 7 as 7.0. The resulting quotient will be 0.875. Remember that the instructions require you to round to the nearest hundredths place. The digit in the thousandths place will be 5, meaning that you need to round up. The final answer is 0.88.

31. B: The answer is 4.43. To solve this problem, you must know how to convert mixed numbers into decimals. Perhaps the easiest way to perform this operation is to convert the mixed number into an improper fraction and then divide the numerator by the denominator. Convert the mixed number into an improper fraction by multiplying the whole number by the denominator and adding the product to the numerator: $4 \times 7 + 3 = 31$, so the improper fraction is $\frac{31}{7}$. Next divide 31 by 7, according to the same procedure used in problems 7 and 8. Remember that when you have to add 0 to 31 in order to continue your calculations, you must put a decimal point directly above in the quotient. Also, since the problem asks you to round to the hundredths place, you must solve the problem to the nearest thousandth.

32. C: The answer is $3\frac{39}{50}$. This problem requires you to understand the conversion of decimals into mixed numbers. 3.78 has value into the hundredths place, so your fraction will have a denominator of 100. There are three whole units and seventy-eight hundredths, a mixed number that can be written as

$3\dfrac{78}{100}$. Next, you must simplify this fraction. The only common factor of 78 and 100 is 2; divide both numerator and denominator by 2 to derive the answer, $3\dfrac{39}{50}$. This fraction cannot be simplified any further.

33. C: The answer is $\dfrac{7}{100}$. To solve this problem, you must know how to convert decimals into fractions. Remember that all of the numbers to the right of a decimal point represent values less than one. So, a decimal number such as this will not include any whole numbers when it is converted into a fraction. The 7 is in the hundredths place, so the number is properly expressed as $\dfrac{7}{100}$. The fraction cannot be simplified because 7 and 100 do not share any factors besides one.

34. D: The answer is $2\dfrac{4}{5}$. This problem requires you to understand how to convert a decimal into a fraction or, in this case, a mixed number. Because there are values to the left of the decimal point, you can tell that this number will be equivalent to a mixed number. Indeed, the number 2.80 is equivalent to $2\dfrac{80}{100}$. Next, list the factors of 80 (1, 2, 4, 5, 8, 10, 16, 20, 40, 80) and 100 (1, 2, 4, 5, 10, 20, 25, 50, 100). The greatest common factor is 20, so divide both numerator and denominator by 20 to derive the simplest form of the fraction, $2\dfrac{4}{5}$.

35. B: The answer is 4:7. To solve this problem, you must know how to convert fractions into ratios. A ratio expresses the relationship between two numbers. For instance, the ratio 2:3 suggests that for every 2 of one thing, there will be 3 of the other. If we applied this ratio to the length and width of a rectangle, for instance, we would be saying that for every 2 units of length, the rectangle must have 3 units of width. A fraction is just one way to express a ratio: The fraction $\dfrac{8}{14}$ is equivalent to the ratio 8:14. To simplify the ratio, divide both sides by the greatest common factor, 2. The simplest form of this ratio is 4:7.

36. B: The answer is 9. This problem requires you to understand how to approach word problems involving fractions and ratios. You are given the total number of students in the class and the fraction of students who are boys: With this information, you can determine the number of boys by multiplying $\dfrac{2}{3}$ by 27. You will find that there are 18 boys in the class. You can then find the number of girls by subtracting the number of boys from the total number of students: 27 – 18 = 9. There are nine girls in the class.

37. A: The answer is 16. To solve this problem, you must understand proportions. A proportion is a comparison between two or more equivalent ratios. A simple proportion is 1:2 :: 2:4, which can be expressed in words as "1 is to 2 as 2 is to 4." Just as 2 is twice 1, 4 is twice 2. Problem 37 asks you to identify a missing term in a proportion. One way to do this is to set up the problem as a set of equivalent fractions and solve for the variable: $\dfrac{3}{2} = \dfrac{24}{x}$. To solve this equation, cross-multiply. You will end up with $3x = 48$. To find the value of x, divide both sides by 3.

38. C: The answer is 24. This problem requires you to understand proportions. You can use the same procedure to solve this problem as you used to solve problem 37. Set up the proportion in the same way as a pair of equivalent fractions: $\frac{7}{42} = \frac{4}{x}$. Then solve for x. To do this, you must cross-multiply (producing $7x = 168$), and then divide both sides by 7. Your calculations should determine that $x = 24$.

39. B: The answer is 64%. To solve this problem, you must know how to convert a decimal into a percent. A percentage is a number expressed in terms of hundredths. When we say, for instance, that a candidate received 55% of the vote, we mean that she received 55 out of every 100 votes cast. When we say that the sales tax is 6%, we mean that for every 100 cents in the price another 6 cents are added to the final cost. To convert a decimal into a percentage, multiply it by 100 or just shift the decimal point two places to the right. In this case, by moving the decimal point two places to the right you can derive the correct answer, 64%.

40. A: The answer is 0.0026%. This problem requires you to understand the conversion of decimals into percentages. Remember that percent is equivalent to quantity out of a hundred; 75%, for instance, is 75 out of 100. To convert a decimal into a percentage, then, multiply the given decimal by 100. A simple way to perform this calculation is to shift the decimal point two places to the right. So for this problem, 0.000026 is equivalent to 0.0026%.

41. D: The answer is 0.38. To solve this problem, you must know how to convert percentages into decimals. This is done by shifting the decimal point two places to the right. This operation is the same as dividing the percentage by 100. In this problem, assume that the decimal is after the eight in 38%. The equivalent decimal, then, is 0.38.

42. C: The answer is 0.176. This problem requires you to understand the conversion of percentages into decimals. A percentage is an amount out of 100; 17.6%, then, is equivalent to 17.6 out of 100, or $\frac{17.6}{100}$. A percentage can be converted into decimal form by dividing it by 100, or, more simply, by shifting the decimal point two places to the left. Therefore, 17.6% is equivalent to 0.176.

43. D: The answer is 1.26. To solve this problem, you must know how to convert percentages into decimals. Remember that a percentage is really just an expression of a value in terms of hundredths. That is, 25% is the same as 25 out of 100. To convert a percentage into a decimal, shift the decimal point two places to the left. In this case, the decimal point is assumed to be after the six in 126%. By shifting the decimal point two places to the left, you find that the equivalent decimal is 1.26.

44. C: The answer is 22%. This problem requires you to understand how to convert fractions into percentages. To do so, divide the numerator by the denominator. This requires placing a decimal point and 0 after the 2. Remember that the instructions ask you to round your quotient to the nearest whole number. The quotient will be an endlessly repeating 0.2, which means that you will round down to 22%. You only need to solve this equation to the thousandths place in order to obtain sufficient information to answer the question.

45. B: The answer is 69%. To solve this problem, you must know how to convert fractions into percentages. This is done by dividing the numerator by the denominator. In this case, the problem is set up as $13\overline{)9.0}$, because a decimal point and 0 are required to make the calculation possible. Although the decimal point is there, you should still treat 9.0 as if it were 90 when performing your division. Since 13 will go into 90 six times, you can place a 6 above the 0 in 9.0. Remember that your quotient will have a

decimal point in the identical place; that is, directly to the left of the 6. If you continue your calculations, you will derive an answer of 0.692... However, once you derive that first 6, you should be able to select the correct answer choice. Remember that percentage is the same as hundredths; in other words, 69% is the same as sixty-nine hundredths.

46. B: The answer is 25%. This problem requires you to understand how to convert fractions into percentages. One way to make this conversion is to divide 17 by 68, which will create a decimal quotient, and then convert this decimal into a percentage. The procedure for division is the same as was used in problem 45; simply divide the numerator (17) by the denominator (68). In order to do so, you will have to express 17 as 17.0. Take the resulting quotient, 0.25, and convert it into a percentage by multiplying it by a hundred or simply shifting the decimal point two places to the right. Of course, you may skip this last step if your quotient makes the right answer apparent. In this problem, for instance, a quotient of 0.25 suggests that only answer choice B can be correct.

47. C: The answer is 59%. To solve this problem, you must know how to convert a fraction into a percentage. Gerald made 13 out of 22 shots, a performance that can also be expressed by the fraction 13/22. To convert this fraction into a percentage, divide the numerator by the denominator: $22 \overline{)13}$. Once you derive the initial 5 in the quotient, you can be fairly certain that answer choice C is correct. Whenever possible, try to take these kinds of shortcuts to save yourself some time. Although the HESI exam gives you plenty of time to complete all of the questions, by saving a little time here and there you can give yourself more opportunities to work through the harder problems.

48. A: The answer is 108. This problem requires you to understand how to find equivalencies involving percentages. One way to solve this problem is to set up the equation $\frac{18}{100} = \frac{x}{600}$. In words, this equation states that 18 out of 100 is equal to some unknown amount out of 600. The first step in solving such an equation is to cross-multiply; in other words, $18 \times 600 = 100x$. This produces $10,800 = 100x$, a problem that can be solved for x by dividing both sides by 100. This calculation shows that $x = 108$, meaning that 108 is 18% of 600.

49. D: The answer is 2.0. To solve this problem, you must know how to find equivalencies involving percentages. This problem can be solved with the same strategy used in problem 48. To begin with, set up the following equation: $\frac{6.4}{100} = \frac{x}{32}$. Next cross-multiply: $6.4 \times 32 = 100x$. This produces $204.8 = 100x$, which is solved for x by dividing both sides of the equation by 100. The value of x is 2.048, which is rounded to 2.0.

50. B: The answer is 17. This problem requires you to know about Roman numerals. This system of numeration is still used in a number of professional contexts. The Roman numerals are as follows: I (1), V (5), X (10), L (50), C (100), D (500), and M (1000). You may also see the lowercase versions of these letters used. The order of the numerals is typically largest to smallest. However, when a smaller number is placed in front of a larger one, the smaller number is to be subtracted from the larger one that follows. For instance, the Roman numeral XIV is 14, as the 1 (I) is to be subtracted from the 5 (V). If the number had been written XVI, it would represent 16, as the 1 (I) is to be added to the 5 (V).

Biology Questions

1. If an organism is *AaBb*, which of the following combinations in the gametes is impossible?
   a. AB

b. aa

c. aB

d. Ab

2. What is the typical result of mitosis in humans?
    a. two diploid cells
    b. two haploid cells
    c. four diploid cells
    d. four haploid cells

3. How does water affect the temperature of a living thing?
    a. Water increases temperature.
    b. Water keeps temperature stable.
    c. Water decreases temperature.
    d. Water does not affect temperature.

4. Which of the following is *not* a product of the Krebs cycle?
    a. carbon dioxide
    b. oxygen
    c. adenosine triphosphate (ATP)
    d. energy carriers

5. What kind of bond connects sugar and phosphate in DNA?
    a. hydrogen
    b. ionic
    c. covalent
    d. overt

6. What is the second part of an organism's scientific name?
    a. species
    b. phylum
    c. population
    d. kingdom

7. How are lipids different than other organic molecules?
    a. They are indivisible.
    b. They are not water soluble.
    c. They contain zinc.
    d. They form long proteins.

8. Which of the following is *not* a steroid?
    a. cholesterol
    b. estrogen
    c. testosterone
    d. hemoglobin

9. Which of the following properties is responsible for the passage of water through a plant?
    a. cohesion
    b. adhesion
    c. osmosis
    d. evaporation

10. Which hormone is produced by the pineal gland?
    a. insulin
    b. testosterone
    c. melatonin
    d. epinephrine

11. What is the name of the organelle that organizes protein synthesis?
    a. mitochondrion
    b. nucleus
    c. ribosome
    d. vacuole

12. During which phase is the chromosome number reduced from diploid to haploid?
    a. S phase
    b. interphase
    c. mitosis
    d. meiosis I

13. What is the name for a cell that does *not* contain a nucleus?
    a. eukaryote
    b. bacteria
    c. prokaryote
    d. cancer

14. What is the name for the physical presentation of an organism's genes?
    a. phenotype
    b. species
    c. phylum
    d. genotype

15. Which of the following forms of water is the densest?
    a. liquid
    b. steam
    c. ice
    d. All forms of water have the same density.

16. What is the longest phase in the life of a cell?
    a. prophase
    b. interphase
    c. anaphase
    d. metaphase

17. Which of the following is *not* found within a bacterial cell?
    a. mitochondria
    b. DNA
    c. vesicles
    d. ribosome

18. Which of the following is a protein?
    a. cellulose

b. hemoglobin

c. estrogen

d. ATP

19. Which of the following structures is *not* involved in translation?

    a. tRNA

    b. mRNA

    c. ribosome

    d. DNA

20. Which of the following is necessary for cell diffusion?

    a. water

    b. membrane

    c. ATP

    d. gradient

21. How many different types of nucleotides are there in DNA?

    a. one

    b. two

    c. four

    d. eight

22. Which of the following cell types has no nucleus?

    a. platelet

    b. red blood cell

    c. white blood cell

    d. phagocyte

23. Which part of aerobic respiration uses oxygen?

    a. osmosis

    b. Krebs cycle

    c. glycolysis

    d. electron transport system

24. Which of the following is the most general taxonomic category?

    a. kingdom

    b. phylum

    c. genus

    d. order

25. What is the name of the process by which a bacterial cell splits into two new cells?

    a. mitosis

    b. meiosis

    c. replication

    d. fission

Biology Answer Key and Explanations

1. B: It is impossible for an *AaBb* organism to have the *aa* combination in the gametes. It is impossible for each letter to be used more than one time, so it would be impossible for the lowercase *a* to appear twice

in the gametes. It would be possible, however, for *Aa* to appear in the gametes, since there is one uppercase *A* and one lowercase *a*. Gametes are the cells involved in sexual reproduction. They are germ cells.

2. A: The typical result of mitosis in humans is two diploid cells. *Mitosis* is the division of a body cell into two daughter cells. Each of the two produced cells has the same set of chromosomes as the parent. A diploid cell contains both sets of homologous chromosomes. A haploid cell contains only one set of chromosomes, which means that it only has a single set of genes. For the HESI exam, you will need to know about all the different stages of cell division for both human and plant cells.

3. B: Water stabilizes the temperature of living things. The ability of warm-blooded animals, including human beings, to maintain a constant internal temperature is known as *homeostasis*. Homeostasis depends on the presence of water in the body. Water tends to minimize changes in temperature because it takes a while to heat up or cool down. When the human body gets warm, the blood vessels dilate and blood moves away from the torso and toward the extremities. When the body gets cold, blood concentrates in the torso. This is the reason why hands and feet tend to get especially cold in cold weather. The HESI exam will require you to understand the basic processes of the human body.

4. B: Oxygen is not one of the products of the Krebs cycle. The *Krebs cycle* is the second stage of cellular respiration. In this stage, a sequence of reactions converts pyruvic acid into carbon dioxide. This stage of cellular respiration produces the phosphate compounds that provide most of the energy for the cell. The Krebs cycle is also known as the citric acid cycle or the tricarboxylic acid cycle. The HESI exam may require you to know all stages of cellular respiration: the process in which a plant cell converts carbon dioxide into oxygen.

5. C: The sugar and phosphate in DNA are connected by covalent bonds. A *covalent bond* is formed when atoms share electrons. It is very common for atoms to share pairs of electrons. An *ionic bond* is created when one or more electrons are transferred between atoms. *Ionic bonds*, also known as *electrovalent bonds*, are formed between ions with opposite charges. There is no such thing as an *overt bond* in chemistry. The HESI exam will require you to understand and have some examples of these different types of bonds.

6. A: The second part of an organism's scientific name is its species. The system of naming species is called binomial nomenclature. The first name is the *genus*, and the second name is the *species*. In binomial nomenclature, species is the most specific designation. This system enables the same name to be used all around the world, so that scientists can communicate with one another. Genus and species are just two of the categories in biological classification, otherwise known as taxonomy. The levels of classification, from most general to most specific, are kingdom, phylum, class, order, family, genus, and species. As you can see, binomial nomenclature only includes the two most specific categories.

7. B: Unlike other organic molecules, lipids are not water soluble. Lipids are typically composed of carbon and hydrogen. Three common types of lipid are fats, waxes, and oils. Indeed, lipids usually feel oily when you touch them. All living cells are primarily composed of lipids, carbohydrates, and proteins. Some examples of fats are lard, corn oil, and butter. Some examples of waxes are beeswax and carnauba wax. Some examples of steroids are cholesterol and ergosterol.

8. D: *Hemoglobin* is not a steroid. It is a protein that helps to move oxygen from the lungs to the various body tissues. Steroids can be either synthetic chemicals used to reduce swelling and inflammation or sex hormones produced by the body. *Cholesterol* is the most abundant steroid in the human body. It is necessary for the creation of bile, though it can be dangerous if the levels in the body become too high. *Estrogen* is a female steroid produced by the ovaries (in females), testes (in males), placenta, and adrenal

cortex. It contributes to adolescent sexual development, menstruation, mood, lactation, and aging. *Testosterone* is the main hormone produced by the testes; it is responsible for the development of adult male sex characteristics.

9. A: The property of cohesion is responsible for the passage of water through a plant. *Cohesion* is the attractive force between two molecules of the same substance. The water in the roots of the plant is drawn upward into the stem, leaves, and flowers by the presence of other water molecules. *Adhesion* is the attractive force between molecules of different substances. *Osmosis* is a process in which water diffuses through a selectively permeable membrane. *Evaporation* is the conversion of water from a liquid to a gas.

10. C: *Melatonin* is produced by the pineal gland. One of the primary functions of melatonin is regulation of the circadian cycle, which is the rhythm of sleep and wakefulness. *Insulin* helps regulate the amount of glucose in the blood. Without insulin, the body is unable to convert blood sugar into energy. *Testosterone* is the main hormone produced by the testes; it is responsible for the development of adult male sex characteristics. *Epinephrine*, also known as adrenaline, performs a number of functions: It quickens and strengthens the heartbeat and dilates the bronchioles. Epinephrine is one of the hormones secreted when the body senses danger.

11. C: *Ribosomes* are the organelles that organize protein synthesis. A ribosome, composed of RNA and protein, is a tiny structure responsible for putting proteins together. The *mitochondrion* converts chemical energy into a form that is more useful for the functions of the cell. The *nucleus* is the central structure of the cell. It contains the DNA and administrates the functions of the cell. The *vacuole* is a cell organelle in which useful materials (for example, carbohydrates, salts, water, and proteins) are stored.

12. D: During *meiosis I*, the chromosome number is reduced from diploid to haploid. *Interphase* is the period of the cell cycle that occurs in between divisions of the cell. In *meiosis*, the homologous chromosomes in a diploid cell separate, reducing the number of chromosomes in each cell by half. *Mitosis* is the phase of cell division in which the cell nucleus divides. *S phase* is the part of the mitotic cycle in which DNA is synthesized.

13. C: Prokaryotic cells do not contain a nucleus. A *prokaryote* is simply a single-celled organism without a nucleus. It is difficult to identify the structures of a prokaryotic cell, even with a microscope. These cells are usually shaped like a rod, a sphere, or a spiral. A *eukaryote* is an organism containing cells with nuclei. Bacterial cells are prokaryotes, but since there are other kinds of prokaryotes, *bacteria* cannot be the correct answer to this question. *Cancer* cells are malignant, atypical cells that reproduce to the detriment of the organism in which they are located.

14. A: *Phenotype* is the physical presentation of an organism's genes. In other words, the phenotype is the physical characteristics of the organism. Phenotype is often contrasted with *genotype*, the genetic makeup of an organism. The genotype of the organism is not visible in its presentation, although some of the characteristics encoded in the genes have to do with physical presentation. A *phylum* is a group of classes that are closely related. A *species* is a group of like organisms that are capable of breeding together and producing similar offspring.

15. A: Liquid is the densest form of water. Water can exist in three states, depending on temperature. Ranging from coldest to hottest, these states are solid, liquid, and gaseous—or ice, water, and steam. Water freezes at zero degrees Celsius. Although the solidity of ice might lead one to believe that it is the densest form of water, water actually expands about nine percent when it is frozen. This is the reason why ice will float in water. Steam is the least dense form of water.

16. B: *Interphase* is the longest phase in the life of a cell. Interphase occurs between cell divisions. *Prophase* is the initial stage of mitosis. It is also the longest stage. During prophase, the chromosomes become visible, and the centrioles divide and position themselves on either side of the nucleus. *Anaphase* is the third phase of mitosis, in which chromosome pairs divide and take up positions on opposing poles. *Metaphase* is the second stage of mitosis. In it, the chromosomes align themselves across the center of the cell.

17. A: Bacterial cells do not contain *mitochondria*. Bacteria are prokaryotes composed of single cells; their cell walls contain peptidoglycans. The functions normally performed in the mitochondria are performed in the cell membrane of the bacterial cell. *DNA* is the nucleic acid that contains the genetic information of the organism. It is in the shape of a double helix. DNA can reproduce itself and can synthesize RNA. A *vesicle* is a small cavity containing fluid. A *ribosome* is a tiny particle composed of RNA and protein, in which polypeptides are constructed.

18. B: *Hemoglobin* is a protein. Proteins contain carbon, nitrogen, oxygen, and hydrogen. These substances are required for the growth and repair of tissue and the formation of enzymes. Hemoglobin is found in red blood cells and contains iron. It is responsible for carrying oxygen from the lungs to the various body tissues. *Adenosine triphosphate* (ATP) is a compound used by living organisms to store and use energy. *Estrogen* is a steroid hormone that stimulates the development of female sex characteristics. *Cellulose* is a complex carbohydrate that composes the better part of the cell wall.

19. D: Deoxyribonucleic acid (*DNA*) is not involved in translation. *Translation* is the process by which messenger RNA (*mRNA*) messages are decoded into polypeptide chains. Transfer RNA (*tRNA*) is a molecule that moves amino acids into the ribosomes during the synthesis of protein. Messenger RNA carries sets of instructions for the conversion of amino acids into proteins from the RNA to the other parts of the cell. *Ribosomes* are the tiny particles in the cell where proteins are put together. Ribosomes are composed of ribonucleic acid (RNA) and protein.

20. A: Water is required for cell diffusion. Diffusion is the movement of molecules from an area of high concentration to an area of lower concentration. This process takes place in the body in a number of different areas. For instance, nutrients diffuse from partially digested food through the walls of the intestine into the bloodstream. Similarly, oxygen that enters the lungs diffuses into the bloodstream through membranes at the end of the alveoli. In all these cases, the body has evolved special membranes that only allow certain materials through.

21. C: There are four different nucleotides in DNA. *Nucleotides* are monomers of nucleic acids, composed of five-carbon sugars, a phosphate group, and a nitrogenous base. Nucleotides make up both DNA and RNA. They are essential for the recording of an organism's genetic information, which guides the actions of the various cells of the body. Nucleotides are also a crucial component of adenosine triphosphate (ATP), one of the parts of DNA and a chemical that enables metabolism and muscle contractions.

22. B: *Red blood cells* do not have a nucleus. These cells are shaped a little like a doughnut, although the hole in the center is not quite open. The other three types of cell have a nucleus. *Platelets*, which are fragments of cells and are released by the bone marrow, contribute to blood clotting. *White blood cells*, otherwise known as leukocytes, help the body fight disease. A *phagocyte* is a cell that can entirely surround bacteria and other microorganisms. The two most common phagocytes are neutrophils and monocytes, both of which are white blood cells.

23. D: The *electron transport system* enacted during aerobic respiration requires oxygen. This is the last component of biological oxidation. *Osmosis* is the movement of fluid from an area of high concentration through a partially permeable membrane to an area of lower concentration. This process usually stops

when the concentration is the same on either side of the membrane. *Glycolysis* is the initial step in the release of glucose energy. The *Krebs cycle* is the last phase of the process in which cells convert food into energy. It is during this stage that carbon dioxide is produced and hydrogen is extracted from molecules of carbon.

24. A: *Kingdom* is the largest, most expansive taxonomic category. A *genus* is a group of related species, which are capable of breeding and producing similar offspring. In binomial nomenclature, genus is the first name. An *order* is any group of similar families. A *phylum* is any group of closely related classes. The HESI exam requires you to know the name and relative specificity of each taxonomic category. They are listed here in order from most general to most specific: kingdom, phylum, class, order, family, genus, and species.

25. D: *Fission* is the process of a bacterial cell splitting into two new cells. Fission is a form of asexual reproduction in which an organism divides into two components; each of these two parts will develop into a distinct organism. The two cells, known as daughter cells, are identical. *Mitosis*, on the other hand, is the part of eukaryotic cell division in which the cell nucleus divides. In *meiosis*, the homologous chromosomes in a diploid cell separate, reducing the number of chromosomes in each cell by half. In *replication*, a cell creates duplicate copies of DNA.

Chemistry Questions

1. Which of the following substances allows for the fastest diffusion?
    a. gas
    b. solid
    c. liquid
    d. plasma

2. What is the oxidation number of hydrogen in CaH_2?
    a. +1
    b. −1
    c. 0
    d. +2

3. Which of the following does *not* exist as a diatomic molecule?
    a. boron
    b. fluorine
    c. oxygen
    d. nitrogen

4. What is another name for aqueous HI?
    a. hydroiodate acid
    b. hydrogen monoiodide
    c. hydrogen iodide
    d. hydriodic acid

5. Which of the following could be an empirical formula?
    a. C4H8
    b. C2H6
    c. CH
    d. C3H6

6. What is the name for the reactant that is entirely consumed by the reaction?
    a. limiting reactant
    b. reducing agent
    c. reaction intermediate
    d. reagent

7. What is the name for the horizontal rows of the periodic table?
    a. groups
    b. periods
    c. families
    d. sets

8. What is the mass (in grams) of 7.35 mol water?
    a. 10.7 g
    b. 18 g
    c. 132 g
    d. 180.6 g

9. Which of the following orbitals is the last to fill?
    a. 1s
    b. 3s
    c. 4p
    d. 6s

10. What is the name of the binary molecular compound NO_5?
    a. nitro pentoxide
    b. ammonium pentoxide
    c. nitrogen pentoxide
    d. pentnitrogen oxide

11. What is the mass (in grams) of 1.0 mol oxygen gas?
    a. 12 g
    b. 16 g
    c. 28 g
    d. 32 g

12. Which kind of radiation has no charge?
    a. beta
    b. alpha
    c. delta
    d. gamma

13. What is the name of the state in which forward and reverse chemical reactions are occurring at the same rate?
    a. equilibrium
    b. constancy
    c. stability
    d. toxicity

14. What is 119°K in degrees Celsius?

a. 32°C
b. −154°C
c. 154°C
d. −32°C

15. What is the SI unit of energy?
   a. ohm
   b. joule
   c. henry
   d. newton

16. What is the name of the device that separates gaseous ions by their mass-to-charge ratio?
   a. mass spectrometer
   b. interferometer
   c. magnetometer
   d. capacitance meter

17. Which material has the smallest specific heat?
   a. water
   b. wood
   c. aluminum
   d. glass

18. What is the name for a reaction in which electrons are transferred from one atom to another?
   a. combustion reaction
   b. synthesis reaction
   c. redox reaction
   d. double-displacement reaction

19. What are van der Waals forces?
   a. the weak forces of attraction between two molecules
   b. the strong forces of attraction between two molecules
   c. hydrogen bonds
   d. conjugal bonds

20. Which of the following gases effuses the fastest?
   a. Cl_2
   b. O_2
   c. N_2
   d. H_2

21. Which of the following elements is *not* involved in many hydrogen bonds?
   a. fluorine
   b. carbon
   c. oxygen
   d. nitrogen

22. What is the mass (in grams) of 0.350 mol copper?
   a. 12.5 g
   b. 14.6 g
   c. 18.5 g

d. 22.2 g

23. How many d orbitals are there in a d subshell?
    a. 5
    b. 7
    c. 9
    d. 11

24. What is the name for the number of protons in an atom?
    a. atomic identity
    b. atomic mass
    c. atomic weight
    d. atomic number

25. Which of the following elements is an alkali metal?
    a. magnesium
    b. rubidium
    c. hydrogen
    d. chlorine

Chemistry Answer Key and Explanations

1. A: Diffusion is fastest through gases. The next fastest medium for diffusion is liquid, followed by plasma, and then solids. In chemistry, diffusion is defined as the movement of matter by the random motions of molecules. In a gas or a liquid, the molecules are in perpetual motion. For instance, in a quantity of seemingly immobile air, molecules of nitrogen and oxygen are constantly bouncing off each other. There is even some miniscule degree of diffusion in solids, which rises in proportion to the temperature of the substance.

2. B: The oxidation number of the hydrogen in CaH_2 is –1. The oxidation number is the positive or negative charge of a monoatomic ion. In other words, the oxidation number is the numerical charge on an ion. An ion is a charged version of an element. Oxidation number is often referred to as oxidation state. Oxidation number is sometimes used to describe the number of electrons that must be added or removed from an atom in order to convert the atom to its elemental form.

3. A: Boron does not exist as a diatomic molecule. The other possible answer choices, fluorine, oxygen, and nitrogen, all exist as diatomic molecules. A diatomic molecule always appears in nature as a pair: The word *diatomic* means "having two atoms." With the exception of astatine, all of the halogens are diatomic. Chemistry students often use the mnemonic BrINClHOF (pronounced "brinkelhoff") to remember all of the diatomic elements: bromine, iodine, nitrogen, chlorine, hydrogen, oxygen, and fluorine. Note that not all of these diatomic elements are halogens.

4. D: Hydriodic acid is another name for aqueous HI. In an aqueous solution, the solvent is water. Hydriodic acid is a polyatomic ion, meaning that it is composed of two or more elements. When this solution has an increased amount of oxygen, the *-ate* suffix on the first word is converted to *-ic*. The HESI exam will require you to know the fundamentals of naming chemicals. This process can be quite complex, so you should carefully review this material before your exam.

5. C: CH could be an empirical formula. An empirical formula is the smallest expression of a chemical formula. To be empirical, a formula must be incapable of being reduced. For this reason, answer choices A,

B, and D are incorrect, as they could all be reduced to a simpler form. Note that empirical formulas are not the same as compounds, which do not have to be irreducible. Two compounds can have the same empirical formula but different molecular formulas. The molecular formula is the actual number of atoms in the molecule.

6. A: A limiting reactant is entirely used up by the chemical reaction. Limiting reactants control the extent of the reaction and determine the quantity of the product. A reducing agent is a substance that reduces the amount of another substance by losing electrons. A reagent is any substance used in a chemical reaction. Some of the most common reagents in the laboratory are sodium hydroxide and hydrochloric acid. The behavior and properties of these substances are known, so they can be effectively used to produce predictable reactions in an experiment.

7. B: The horizontal rows of the periodic table are called periods. The vertical columns of the periodic table are known as groups or families. All of the elements in a group have similar properties. The relationships between the elements in each period are similar as you move from left to right. The periodic table was developed by Dmitri Mendeleev to organize the known elements according to their similarities. New elements can be added to the periodic table without necessitating a redesign.

8. C: The mass of 7.35 mol water is 132 grams. You should be able to find the mass of various chemical compounds when you are given the number of mols. The information required to perform this function is included on the periodic table. To solve this problem, find the molecular mass of water by finding the respective weights of hydrogen and oxygen. Remember that water contains two hydrogen molecules and one oxygen molecule. The molecular mass of hydrogen is roughly 1, and the molecular mass of oxygen is roughly 16. A molecule of water, then, has approximately 18 grams of mass. Multiply this by 7.35 mol, and you will obtain the answer 132.3, which is closest to answer choice C.

9. D: Of these orbitals, the last to fill is 6s. Orbitals fill in the following order: 1s, 2s, 2p, 3s, 3p, 4s, 3d, 4p, 5s, 4d, 5p, 6s, 4f, 5d, 6p, 7s, 5f, 6d, and 7p. The number is the orbital number, and the letter is the sublevel identification. Sublevel s has one orbital and can hold a maximum of two electrons. Sublevel p has three orbitals and can hold a maximum of six electrons. Sublevel d has five orbitals and can hold a maximum of 10 electrons. Sublevel f has seven orbitals and can hold a maximum of 14 electrons.

10. C: Nitrogen pentoxide is the name of the binary molecular compound NO_5. The format given in answer choice C is appropriate when dealing with two nonmetals. A prefix is used to denote the number of atoms of each element. Note that when there are seven atoms of a given element, the prefix *hepta-* is used instead of the usual *septa-*. Also, when the first atom in this kind of binary molecular compound is single, it does not need to be given the prefix *mono-*.

11. D: The mass of 1.0 mol oxygen gas is 32 grams. The molar mass of oxygen can be obtained from the periodic table. In most versions of the table, the molar mass of the element is directly beneath the full name of the element. There is a little trick to this question. Oxygen is a diatomic molecule, which means that it always appears in pairs. In order to determine the mass in grams of 1.0 mol of oxygen gas, then, you must double the molar mass. The listed mass is 16, so the correct answer to the problem is 32.

12. D: Gamma radiation has no charge. This form of electromagnetic radiation can travel a long distance and can penetrate the human body. Sunlight and radio waves are both examples of gamma radiation. Alpha radiation has a 2+ charge. It only travels short distances and cannot penetrate clothing or skin. Radium and uranium both emit alpha radiation. Beta radiation has a 1– charge. It can travel several feet through the air and is capable of penetrating the skin. This kind of radiation can be damaging to health over a long period of exposure. There is no such thing as delta radiation.

13. A: When forward and reverse chemical reactions are taking place at the same rate, a chemical reaction has achieved equilibrium. This means that the respective concentrations of reactants and products do not change over time. In theory, a chemical reaction will remain in equilibrium indefinitely. One of the common tasks in the chemistry lab is to find the equilibrium constant (or set of relative concentrations that result in equilibrium) for a given reaction. In thermal equilibrium, there is no net heat exchange between a body and its surroundings. In dynamic equilibrium, any motion in one direction is offset by an equal motion in the other direction.

14. B: 119°K is equivalent to –154 degrees Celsius. It is likely that you will have to perform at least one temperature conversion on the HESI exam. To convert degrees Kelvin to degrees Celsius, simply subtract 273. To convert degrees Celsius to degrees Kelvin, simply add 273. To convert degrees Kelvin into degrees Fahrenheit, multiply by 9/5 and subtract 460. To convert degrees Fahrenheit to degrees Kelvin, add 460 and then multiply by 5/9. To convert degrees Celsius to degrees Fahrenheit, multiply by 9/5 and then add 32. To convert degrees Fahrenheit to degrees Celsius, subtract 32 and then multiply by 5/9.

15. B: The *joule* is the SI unit of energy. Energy is the ability to do work or generate heat. In regard to electrical energy, a joule is the amount of electrical energy required to pass a current of one ampere through a resistance of one ohm for one second. In physical or mechanical terms, the joule is the amount of energy required for a force of one newton to act over a distance of one meter. The *ohm* is a unit of electrical resistance. The *henry* is a unit of inductance. The *newton* is a unit of force.

16. A: A *mass spectrometer* separates gaseous ions according to their mass-to-charge ratio. This machine is used to distinguish the various elements in a piece of matter. An *interferometer* measures the wavelength of light by comparing the interference phenomena of two waves: an experimental wave and a reference wave. A *magnetometer* measures the direction and magnitude of a magnetic field. Finally, a *capacitance meter* measures the capacitance of a capacitor. Some sophisticated capacitance meters may also measure inductance, leakage, and equivalent series resistance.

17. C: Of the given materials, aluminum has the smallest specific heat. The specific heat of a substance is the amount of heat required to raise the temperature of one gram of the substance by one degree Celsius. In some cases, specific heat is expressed as a ratio of the heat required to raise the temperature of one gram of a substance by one degree Celsius to the heat required to raise the temperature of one gram of water by one degree Celsius.

18. C: In a *redox* reaction, also known as an oxidation-reduction reaction, electrons are transferred from one atom to another. A redox reaction changes the oxidation numbers of the atoms. In a *combustion* reaction, one material combines with an oxidizer to form a product and generate heat. In a *synthesis* reaction, multiple chemicals are combined to create a more complex product. In a *double-displacement* reaction, two chemical compounds trade bonds or ions and create two different compounds. Other common chemical reactions you may need to know for the HESI exam are the acid-base reaction, analysis reaction, single-displacement reaction, isomerization reaction, and hydrolysis reaction.

19. A: Van der Waals forces are the weak forces of attraction between two molecules. The van der Waals force is considered to be any of the attractive or repulsive forces between electrons that are not related to electrostatic interaction or covalent bonds. Compared to other chemical bonds, the strength of van der Waals forces is small. However, these forces have a great effect on a substance's solubility and other characteristics. The HESI exam may require you to demonstrate knowledge of all the major chemical forces.

20. D: Of the given gases, H_2 effuses the fastest. It has the smallest molecular weight, and it is therefore capable of moving faster than the molecules represented by the other answer choices. In chemistry,

effusion is defined as the flow of a gas through a small opening. The rate of effusion of a substance is inversely proportional to the square root of the density of the substance. This means that the less dense a substance is, the faster it will effuse. This agrees with the common observation that thick smoke tends to linger in the same form for a longer period than thin smoke or steam.

21. B: Carbon is not involved in many hydrogen bonds. A hydrogen bond occurs when an atom of hydrogen that has a covalent bond with an electronegative atom forms a bond with a third atom. The original covalent bond involving hydrogen gives away protons, and the third element receives them. One of the reasons that fluorine, oxygen, and nitrogen are frequently part of a hydrogen bond is that they have a strong electronegativity and are therefore able to form more durable bonds. Chlorine is another element frequently involved in hydrogen bonds.

22. D: The mass of 0.350 mol copper is 22.2 grams. This problem requires the use of the periodic table. There you will see that the molecular mass of copper is approximately 63.5. Take this figure and multiply it by the amount of copper given by the question: 0.350 mol. The resulting figure is 22.225, which, rounded to the nearest tenth, is 22.2 grams. In order to succeed on the HESI exam, you will need to be able to perform these simple calculations of mass.

23. A: There are five d orbitals in a d subshell (or sublevel). Each of these orbitals can hold two electrons, so sublevel d is capable of holding 10 electrons. The s subshell has one orbital, the p subshell has three orbitals, the d subshell has five orbitals, and the f subshell has seven orbitals. In chemistry, the electron configuration of an atom is expressed in the following form, using helium as an example: $1s^2$. In this notation, the 1 indicates that the electrons are found in the first energy level of the atom, the s indicates that the electrons are in a spherical orbit, and the superscript 2 indicates that there are 2 total electrons in the first energy level subshell.

24. D: The number of protons in an atom is the atomic number. Protons are the fundamental positive unit of an atom. They are located in the nucleus. In a neutral atom (an atom with neither positive nor negative charge), the number of protons in the nucleus is equal to the number of electrons orbiting the nucleus. When it needs to be expressed, atomic number is written as a subscript in front of the element's symbol, for example in $_{13}$Al. Atomic mass, meanwhile, is the average mass of the various isotopes of a given element. Atomic identity and atomic weight are not concepts in chemistry.

25. B: Rubidium is an alkali metal. The alkali metals are located in group 1 of the periodic table. These soft substances melt at a low temperature and are typically white in color. The alkali metals are lithium, sodium, potassium, rubidium, cesium, and francium. Rubidium, cesium, and francium are not commonly encountered in the natural world. The alkali metals are highly reactive, meaning that they easily engage in chemical reactions when combined with other elements. These metals have a low density and tend to react violently with water.

Anatomy and Physiology Questions

1. What is the name of the structure that prevents food from entering the airway?
   a. trachea
   b. esophagus
   c. diaphragm
   d. epiglottis

2. Which substance makes up the pads that provide support between the vertebrae?
   a. bone

b. cartilage
c. tendon
d. fat

3. How many different types of tissue are there in the human body?
   a. four
   b. six
   c. eight
   d. ten

4. What is the name of the outermost layer of skin?
   a. dermis
   b. epidermis
   c. subcutaneous tissue
   d. hypodermis

5. Which hormone stimulates milk production in the breasts during lactation?
   a. norepinephrine
   b. antidiuretic hormone
   c. prolactin
   d. oxytocin

6. Which of the following structures has the lowest blood pressure?
   a. arteries
   b. arteriole
   c. venule
   d. vein

7. Which of the heart chambers is the most muscular?
   a. left atrium
   b. right atrium
   c. left ventricle
   d. right ventricle

8. Which part of the brain interprets sensory information?
   a. cerebrum
   b. hindbrain
   c. cerebellum
   d. medulla oblongata

9. Which of the following proteins is produced by cartilage?
   a. actin
   b. estrogen
   c. collagen
   d. myosin

10. Which component of the nervous system is responsible for lowering the heart rate?
    a. central nervous system
    b. sympathetic nervous system
    c. parasympathetic nervous system
    d. distal nervous system

11. Which type of substance breaks down to form urea?
    a. lipid
    b. protein
    c. carbohydrate
    d. iron

12. What is the name for a joint that can only move in two directions?
    a. hinge
    b. insertion
    c. ball and socket
    d. flange

13. In which of the following muscle types are the filaments arranged in a disorderly manner?
    a. cardiac
    b. smooth
    c. skeletal
    d. rough

14. How much air does an adult inhale in an average breath?
    a. 500 mL
    b. 750 mL
    c. 1000 mL
    d. 1250 mL

15. Which type of cell secretes antibodies?
    a. bacterial cell
    b. viral cell
    c. lymph cell
    d. plasma cells

16. Which force motivates filtration in the kidneys?
    a. osmosis
    b. smooth muscle contraction
    c. peristalsis
    d. blood pressure

17. Which of the following hormones decreases the concentration of blood glucose?
    a. insulin
    b. glucagon
    c. growth hormone
    d. glucocorticoids

18. Which structure controls the hormones secreted by the pituitary gland?
    a. hypothalamus
    b. adrenal gland
    c. testes
    d. pancreas

19. How much of a female's blood volume is composed of red blood cells?
    a. 10%

b. 25%
c. 40%
d. 70%

20. Which type of cholesterol is considered to be the best for health?
    a. LDL
    b. HDL
    c. VLDL
    d. VHDL

21. Where are the vocal cords located?
    a. bronchi
    b. trachea
    c. larynx
    d. epiglottis

22. Where does gas exchange occur in the human body?
    a. alveoli
    b. bronchi
    c. larynx
    d. pharynx

23. Which structure of the nervous system carries action potential in the direction of a synapse?
    a. cell body
    b. axon
    c. neuron
    d. myelin

24. Where is the parathyroid gland located?
    a. neck
    b. back
    c. side
    d. brain

25. What is the name of the process in the lungs by which oxygen is transported from the air to the blood?
    a. osmosis
    b. diffusion
    c. dissipation
    d. reverse osmosis

Anatomy and Physiology Answer Key and Explanations

1. D: The epiglottis covers the trachea during swallowing, thus preventing food from entering the airway. The trachea, also known as the windpipe, is a cylindrical portion of the respiratory tract that joins the larynx with the lungs. The esophagus connects the throat and the stomach. When a person swallows, the esophagus contracts to force the food down into the stomach. Like other structures in the respiratory system, the esophagus secretes mucus for lubrication.

2. B: The pads that support the vertebrae are made up of cartilage. Cartilage, a strong form of connective tissue, cushions and supports the joints. Cartilage also makes up the larynx and the outer ear. Bone is a

form of connective tissue that comprises the better part of the skeleton. It includes both organic and inorganic substances. Tendons connect the muscles to other structures of the body, typically bones. Tendons can increase and decrease in length as the bones move. Fat is a combination of lipids; in humans, fat forms a layer beneath the skin and on the outside of the internal organs.

3. A: There are four different types of tissue in the human body: epithelial, connective, muscle, and nerve. *Epithelial* tissue lines the internal and external surfaces of the body. It is like a sheet, consisting of squamous, cuboidal, and columnar cells. They can expand and contract, like on the inner lining of the bladder. *Connective* tissue provides the structure of the body, as well as the links between various body parts. Tendons, ligaments, cartilage, and bone are all examples of connective tissue. *Muscle* tissue is composed of tiny fibers, which contract to move the skeleton. There are three types of muscle tissue: smooth, cardiac, and skeletal. *Nerve* tissue makes up the nervous system; it is composed of nerve cells, nerve fibers, neuroglia, and dendrites.

4. B: The epidermis is the outermost layer of skin. The thickness of this layer of skin varies over different parts of the body. For instance, the epidermis on the eyelids is very thin, while the epidermis over the soles of the feet is much thicker. The dermis lies directly beneath the epidermis. It is composed of collagen, elastic tissue, and reticular fibers. Beneath the dermis lies the subcutaneous tissue, which consists of fat, blood vessels, and nerves. The subcutaneous tissue contributes to the regulation of body temperature. The hypodermis is the layer of cells underneath the dermis; it is generally considered to be a part of the subcutaneous tissue.

5. C: *Prolactin* stimulates the production of breast milk during lactation. *Norepinephrine* is a hormone and neurotransmitter secreted by the adrenal gland that regulates heart rate, blood pressure, and blood sugar. *Antidiuretic hormone* is produced by the hypothalamus and secreted by the pituitary gland. It regulates the concentration of urine and triggers the contractions of the arteries and capillaries. *Oxytocin* is a hormone secreted by the pituitary gland that makes it easier to eject milk from the breast and manages the contractions of the uterus during labor.

6. D: Of the given structures, veins have the lowest blood pressure. *Veins* carry oxygen-poor blood from the outlying parts of the body to the heart. An *artery* carries oxygen-rich blood from the heart to the peripheral parts of the body. An *arteriole* extends from an artery to a capillary. A *venule* is a tiny vein that extends from a capillary to a larger vein.

7. C: Of the four heart chambers, the left ventricle is the most muscular. When it contracts, it pushes blood out to the organs and extremities of the body. The right ventricle pushes blood into the lungs. The atria, on the other hand, receive blood from the outlying parts of the body and transport it into the ventricles. The basic process works as follows: Oxygen-poor blood fills the right atrium and is pumped into the right ventricle, from which it is pumped into the pulmonary artery and on to the lungs. In the lungs, this blood is oxygenated. The blood then reenters the heart at the left atrium, which when full pumps into the left ventricle. When the left ventricle is full, blood is pushed into the aorta and on to the organs and extremities of the body.

8. A: The *cerebrum* is the part of the brain that interprets sensory information. It is the largest part of the brain. The cerebrum is divided into two hemispheres, connected by a thin band of tissue called the corpus callosum. The *cerebellum* is positioned at the back of the head, between the brain stem and the cerebrum. It controls both voluntary and involuntary movements. The *medulla oblongata* forms the base of the brain. This part of the brain is responsible for blood flow and breathing, among other things.

9. C: *Collagen* is the protein produced by cartilage. Bone, tendon, and cartilage are all mainly composed of collagen. *Actin* and *myosin* are the proteins responsible for muscle contractions. Actin makes up the

- 173 -

thinner fibers in muscle tissue, while myosin makes up the thicker fibers. Myosin is the most numerous cell protein in human muscle. *Estrogen* is one of the steroid hormones produced mainly by the ovaries. Estrogen motivates the menstrual cycle and the development of female sex characteristics.

10. C: The parasympathetic nervous system is responsible for lowering the heart rate. It slows down the heart rate, dilates the blood vessels, and increases the secretions of the digestive system. The central nervous system is composed of the brain and the spinal cord. The sympathetic nervous system is a part of the autonomic nervous system; its role is to oppose the actions taken by the parasympathetic nervous system. So, the sympathetic nervous system accelerates the heart, contracts the blood vessels, and decreases the secretions of the digestive system.

11. B: Urea is formed during the breakdown of proteins. It is a nitrogen-rich substance filtered out of the bloodstream by the kidneys and expelled from the body in the urine. Individuals with an elevated level of urea in their bloodstream may be suffering from kidney failure. In humans and most animals, urea is the primary component of urine. However, urine also contains uric acid and ammonia. Both of these substances can be toxic to humans if they are not expelled from the body. This is one of the dangers of kidney disease and kidney failure.

12. A: A hinge joint can only move in two directions. The elbow is a hinge joint. It can only bring the lower arm closer to the upper arm or move it away from the upper arm. In a ball-and-socket joint, the rounded top of one bone fits into a concave part of another bone, enabling the first bone to rotate around in this socket. This connection is slightly less stable than other types of joints in the human body and is therefore supported by a denser network of ligaments. The shoulder and hip are both examples of ball-and-socket joints.

13: B. Smooth muscle tissue is said to be arranged in a disorderly fashion because it is not striated like the other two types of muscle: cardiac and skeletal. Striations are lines that can only be seen with a microscope. *Smooth* muscle is typically found in the supporting tissues of hollow organs and blood vessels. *Cardiac* muscle is found exclusively in the heart; it is responsible for the contractions that pump blood throughout the body. *Skeletal* muscle, by far the most preponderant in the body, controls the movements of the skeleton. The contractions of skeletal muscle are responsible for all voluntary motion. There is no such thing as *rough* muscle.

14. A: An adult inhales 500 mL of air in an average breath. Interestingly, humans can inhale about eight times as much air in a single breath as they do in an average breath. People tend to take a larger breath after making a larger inhalation. This is one reason that many breathing therapies, for instance those incorporated into yoga practice, focus on making a complete exhalation. The process of respiration is managed by the autonomic nervous system. The body requires a constant replenishing of oxygen, so even brief interruptions in respiration can be damaging or fatal.

15. D: *Plasma* cells secrete antibodies. These cells, also known as plasmacytes, are located in lymphoid tissue. Antibodies are only secreted in response to a particular stimulus, usually the detection of an antigen in the body. Antigens include bacteria, viruses, and parasites. Once released, antibodies bind to the antigen and neutralize it. When faced with a new antigen, the body may require some time to develop appropriate antibodies. Once the body has learned about an antigen, however, it does not forget how to produce the correct antibodies.

16. D: The force of *blood pressure* motivates filtration in the kidneys. *Filtration* is the process through which the kidneys remove waste products from the body. All of the water in the blood passes through the kidneys every 45 minutes. Waste products are diverted into ducts and excreted from the body, while the

healthy components of the water in blood are reabsorbed into the bloodstream. *Peristalsis* is the set of involuntary muscle movements that move food through the digestive system.

17. A: *Insulin* decreases the concentration of blood glucose. It is produced by the pancreas. *Glucagon* is a hormone produced by the pancreas. Glucagon acts in opposition to insulin, motivating an increase in the levels of blood sugar. *Growth hormone* is secreted by the pituitary gland. It is responsible for the growth of the body, specifically by metabolizing proteins, carbohydrates, and lipids. The *glucocorticoids* are a group of steroid hormones that are produced by the adrenal cortex. The glucocorticoids contribute to the metabolism of carbohydrates, proteins, and fats.

18. A: The *hypothalamus* controls the hormones secreted by the pituitary gland. This part of the brain maintains the body temperature and helps to control metabolism. The *adrenal glands*, which lie above the kidneys, secrete steroidal hormones, epinephrine, and norepinephrine. The *testes* are the male reproductive glands, responsible for the production of sperm and testosterone. The *pancreas* secretes insulin and a fluid that aids in digestion.

19. C: Forty percent of female blood volume is composed of red blood cells. Red blood cells, otherwise known as erythrocytes, are large and do not have a nucleus. These cells are produced in the bone marrow and carry oxygen throughout the body. White blood cells, also known as leukocytes, make up about 1% of the blood volume. About 55% of the blood volume is made up of plasma, which itself is primarily composed of water. The plasma in blood supplies cells with nutrients and removes metabolic waste. Blood also contains platelets, otherwise known as thrombocytes, which are essential to effective blood clotting.

20. B: High-density lipoproteins (*HDL*) are considered to be the healthiest form of cholesterol. This type of cholesterol actually reduces the risk of heart disease. A lipoprotein is composed of both lipid and protein. These substances cannot move through the bloodstream by themselves; they must be carried along by some other substance. Although most people think of cholesterol as an unhealthy substance, it helps to maintain cell walls and produce hormones. Cholesterol is also important in the production of vitamin D and the bile acids that aid digestion. The other answer choices are low-density lipoproteins (*LDL*), very-low-density lipoproteins (*VLDL*), and very-high-density lipoproteins (*VHDL*).

21. C: The vocal cords are located in the larynx. These elastic bands vibrate and produce sound when air passes through them. The *larynx* lies between the pharynx and the trachea. The pharynx is the section of the throat that extends from the mouth and the nasal cavities to the larynx, at which point it becomes the esophagus. The *trachea* is the tube running from the larynx down to the lungs, where it terminates in the *bronchi*. The *epiglottis* is the flap that blocks food from the lungs by descending over the trachea during a swallow.

22. A: Gas exchange occurs in the *alveoli*, the minute air sacs on the interior of the lungs. The *bronchi* are large cartilage-based tubes of air; they extend from the end of the trachea into the lungs, where they branch apart. The *larynx*, which houses the vocal cords, is positioned between the trachea and the pharynx; it is involved in swallowing, breathing, and speaking. The *pharynx* extends from the nose to the uppermost portions of the trachea and esophagus. In order to enter these two structures, air and other matter must pass through the pharynx.

23. B: *Axons* carry action potential in the direction of synapses. Axons are the long, fiberlike structures that carry information from neurons. Electrical impulses travel along the body of the axons, some of which are up to a foot long. A *neuron* is a type of cell that is responsible for sending information throughout the body. There are several types of neurons, including muscle neurons, which respond to instructions for movement; sensory neurons, which transmit information about the external world; and

interneurons, which relay messages between neurons. *Myelin* is a fat that coats the nerves and ensures the accurate transmission of information in the nervous system.

24. A: The parathyroid gland is located in the neck, directly behind the thyroid gland. It is responsible for the metabolism of calcium. It is part of the endocrine system. When the supply of calcium in blood diminishes to unhealthy levels, the parathyroid gland motivates the secretion of a hormone that encourages the bones to release calcium into the bloodstream. The parathyroid gland also regulates the amount of phosphate in the blood by stimulating the excretion of phosphates in the urine.

25. B: In the lungs, oxygen is transported from the air to the blood through the process of *diffusion*. Specifically, the alveolar membranes withdraw the oxygen from the air in the lungs into the bloodstream. *Osmosis* is the movement of a solution from an area of low concentration to an area of higher concentration through a permeable membrane. *Dissipation* is any wasteful consumption or use. *Reverse osmosis* is a process for purifying a solution by forcing it through a membrane that blocks only certain pollutants.

Secret Key #1 – Time is Your Greatest Enemy

To succeed on the HESI A² exam, you must use your time wisely. Most students do not finish at least one section.

Success Strategy #1

Pace Yourself

Wear a watch to the HESI A² exam. At the beginning of the test, check the time (or start a chronometer on your watch to count the minutes), and check the time after each passage or every few questions to make sure you are "on schedule."

If you find that you are falling behind time during the test, you must speed up. Even though a rushed answer is more likely to be incorrect, it is better to miss a couple of questions by being rushed, than to completely miss later questions by not having enough time. It is better to end with more time than you need than to run out of time.

If you are forced to speed up, do it efficiently. Usually one or more answer choices can be eliminated without too much difficulty. Above all, don't panic. Don't speed up and just begin guessing at random choices. By pacing yourself, and continually monitoring your progress against your watch, you will always know exactly how far ahead or behind you are with your available time. If you find that you are a few minutes behind on a section, don't skip questions without spending any time on it, just to catch back up. Begin spending a little less time per question and after a few questions, you will have caught back up more gradually. Once you catch back up, you can continue working each problem at your normal pace. If you have time at the end, go back then and finish the questions that you left behind.

Furthermore, don't dwell on the problems that you were rushed on. If a problem was taking up too much time and you made a hurried guess, it must have been difficult. The difficult questions are the ones you are most likely to miss anyway, so it isn't a big loss. If you have time left over, as you review the skipped questions, start at the earliest skipped question, spend at most another minute, and then move on to the next skipped question.

Always mark skipped questions in your workbook, NOT on the Scantron. Last minute guessing will be covered in the next chapter.

Lastly, sometimes it is beneficial to slow down if you are constantly getting ahead of time. You are always more likely to catch a careless mistake by working more slowly than quickly, and among very high-scoring students (those who are likely to have lots of time left over), careless errors affect the score more than mastery of material.

Scanning

Don't waste time reading, enjoying, and completely understanding the passage. Simply scan the passage to get a rough idea of what it is about. You will return to the passage for each question, so there is no need to memorize it. Only spend as much time scanning as is necessary to get a vague impression of its overall subject content.

Secret Key #2 – Guessing is not guesswork.

Most students do not understand the impact that proper guessing can have on their score. Unless you score extremely high, guessing will contribute a significant amount of points to your score.

Monkeys Take the HESI A^2 Exam

What most students don't realize is that to insure that random 25% chance, you have to guess randomly. If you put 20 monkeys in a room to take the HESI A² exam, assuming they answered once per question and behaved themselves, on average they would get 25% of the questions correct. Put 20 students in the room, and the average will be much lower among guessed questions. Why?

1. The HESI A² exam intentionally has deceptive answer choices that "look" right. A student has no idea about a question, so picks the "best looking" answer, which is often wrong. The monkey has no idea what looks good and what doesn't, so will consistently be lucky about 25% of the time.
2. Students will eliminate answer choices from the guessing pool based on a hunch or intuition. Simple but correct answers often get excluded, leaving a 0% chance of being correct. The monkey has no clue, and often gets lucky with the best choice.

This is why the process of elimination endorsed by most test courses is flawed and detrimental to your performance- students don't guess, they make an ignorant stab in the dark that is usually worse than random.

Success Strategy #2

Let me introduce one of the most valuable ideas of this course- the $5 challenge:

You only mark your "best guess" if you are willing to bet $5 on it.
You only eliminate choices from guessing if you are willing to bet $5 on it.

Why $5? Five dollars is an amount of money that is small yet not insignificant, and can really add up fast (20 questions could cost you $100). Likewise, each answer choice on one question of the HESI A² exam will have a small impact on your overall score, but it can really add up to a lot of points in the end.

The process of elimination IS valuable. The following shows your chance of guessing it right:

If you eliminate this many choices:	0
0	25%
1	33%
2	50%
3	100%

However, if you accidentally eliminate the right answer or go on a hunch for an incorrect answer, your chances drop dramatically: to 0%. By guessing among all the answer choices, you are GUARANTEED to have a shot at the right answer.

That's why the $5 test is so valuable- if you give up the advantage and safety of a pure guess, it had better be worth the risk.

What we still haven't covered is how to be sure that whatever guess you make is truly random. Here's the easiest way:

Always pick the first answer choice among those remaining.

Such a technique means that you have decided, **before you see a single test question**, exactly how you are going to guess- and since the order of choices tells you nothing about which one is correct, this guessing technique is perfectly random.

Specific Guessing Techniques

Similar Answer Choices
When you have two answer choices that are direct opposites, one of them is usually the correct answer. Example:
A.) forward
B.) backward

These two answer choices are very similar and fall into the same family of answer choices. A family of answer choices is when two or three answer choices are very similar. Often two will be opposites and one may show an equality.
Example:
A.) excited
B.) overjoyed
C.) thrilled
D.) upset

Note how the first three choices are all related. They all ask describe a state of happiness. However, choice D is not in the same family of questions. Being upset is the direct opposite of happiness.

Summary of Guessing Techniques
1. Eliminate as many choices as you can by using the $5 test. Use the common guessing strategies to help in the elimination process, but only eliminate choices that pass the $5 test.
2. Among the remaining choices, only pick your "best guess" if it passes the $5 test.
3. Otherwise, guess randomly by picking the first remaining choice that was not eliminated.

Secret Key #3 – Practice Smarter, Not Harder

Many students delay the test preparation process because they dread the awful amounts of practice time they think necessary to succeed on the test. We have refined an effective method that will take you only a fraction of the time.

There are a number of "obstacles" in your way on the HESI A² exam. Among these are answering questions, finishing in time, and mastering test-taking strategies. All must be executed on the day of the test at peak performance, or your score will suffer. The HESI A² exam is a mental marathon that has a large impact on your future.

Just like a marathon runner, it is important to work your way up to the full challenge. So first you just worry about questions, and then time, and finally strategy:

Success Strategy #3

1. Find a good source for HESI A² exam practice tests.
2. If you are willing to make a larger time investment (or if you want to really "learn" the material, a time consuming but ultimately valuable endeavor), consider buying one of the better study guides on the market
3. Take a practice test with no time constraints, with all study helps "open book." Take your time with questions and focus on applying the strategies.
4. Take another test, this time with time constraints, with all study helps "open book."
5. Take a final practice test with no open material and time limits.

If you have time to take more practice tests, just repeat step 5. By gradually exposing yourself to the full rigors of the test environment, you will condition your mind to the stress of test day and maximize your success.

Secret Key #4 – Prepare, Don't Procrastinate

Let me state an obvious fact: if you take the HESI A² exam three times, you will get three different scores. This is due to the way you feel on test day, the level of preparedness you have, and, despite HESI A² exam's claims to the contrary, some tests WILL be easier for you than others.

Since your acceptance will largely depend on your score, you should maximize your chances of success. In order to maximize the likelihood of success, you've got to prepare in advance. This means taking practice tests and spending time learning the information and test taking strategies you will need to succeed.

Since you have to pay a registration fee each time you take the HESI A² exam, don't take it as a "practice" test. Feel free to take sample tests on your own, but when you go to take the HESI A² exam, be prepared, be focused, and do your best the first time!

Secret Key #5 – Test Yourself

Everyone knows that time is money. There is no need to spend too much of your time or too little of your time preparing for the HESI A² exam. You should only spend as much of your precious time preparing as is necessary for you to pass it.

Success Strategy #5

Once you have taken a practice test under real conditions of time constraints, then you will know if you are ready for the test or not.

If you have scored extremely high the first time that you take the practice test, then there is not much point in spending countless hours studying. You are already there.

Benchmark your abilities by retaking practice tests and seeing how much you have improved. Once you score high enough to get accepted into the school of your choice, then you are ready.

If you have scored well below where you need, then knuckle down and begin studying in earnest. Check your improvement regularly through the use of practice tests under real conditions. Above all, don't worry, panic, or give up. The key is perseverance!

Then, when you go to take the HESI A² exam, remain confident and remember how well you did on the practice tests. If you can score high enough on a practice test, then you can do the same on the real thing.

General Strategies

The most important thing you can do is to ignore your fears and jump into the test immediately- do not be overwhelmed by any strange-sounding terms. You have to jump into the test like jumping into a pool- all at once is the easiest way.

Make Predictions

As you read and understand the question, try to guess what the answer will be. Remember that several of the answer choices are wrong, and once you begin reading them, your mind will immediately become cluttered with answer choices designed to throw you off. Your mind is typically the most focused immediately after you have read the question and digested its contents. If you can, try to predict what the correct answer will be. You may be surprised at what you can predict.

Quickly scan the choices and see if your prediction is in the listed answer choices. If it is, then you can be quite confident that you have the right answer. It still won't hurt to check the other answer choices, but most of the time, you've got it!

Answer the Question

It may seem obvious to only pick answer choices that answer the question, but the test writers can create some excellent answer choices that are wrong. Don't pick an answer just because it sounds right, or you believe it to be true. It MUST answer the question. Once you've made your selection, always go back and check it against the question and make sure that you didn't misread the question, and the answer choice does answer the question posed.

Benchmark

After you read the first answer choice, decide if you think it sounds correct or not. If it doesn't, move on to the next answer choice. If it does, mentally mark that answer choice. This doesn't mean that you've definitely selected it as your answer choice, it just means that it's the best you've seen thus far. Go ahead and read the next choice. If the next choice is worse than the one you've already selected, keep going to the next answer choice. If the next choice is better than the choice you've already selected, mentally mark the new answer choice as your best guess.

The first answer choice that you select becomes your standard. Every other answer choice must be benchmarked against that standard. That choice is correct until proven otherwise by another answer choice beating it out. Once you've decided that no other answer choice seems as good, do one final check to ensure that your answer choice answers the question posed.

Valid Information

Don't discount any of the information provided in the question. Every piece of information may be necessary to determine the correct answer. None of the information in the question is there to throw you off (while the answer choices will certainly have information to throw you off). If two seemingly unrelated topics are discussed, don't ignore either. You can be confident there is a relationship, or it wouldn't be included in the question, and you are probably going to have to determine what is that relationship to find the answer.

Avoid "Fact Traps"

Don't get distracted by a choice that is factually true. Your search is for the answer that answers the question. Stay focused and don't fall for an answer that is true but incorrect. Always go back to the question and make sure you're choosing an answer that actually answers the question and is not just a true statement. An answer can be factually correct, but it MUST answer the question asked. Additionally, two answers can both be seemingly correct, so be sure to read all of the answer choices, and make sure that you get the one that BEST answers the question.

Milk the Question

Some of the questions may throw you completely off. They might deal with a subject you have not been exposed to, or one that you haven't reviewed in years. While your lack of knowledge about the subject will be a hindrance, the question itself can give you many clues that will help you find the correct answer. Read the question carefully and look for clues. Watch particularly for adjectives and nouns describing difficult terms or words that you don't recognize. Regardless of if you completely understand a word or not, replacing it with a synonym either provided or one you more familiar with may help you to understand what the questions are asking. Rather than wracking your mind about specific detailed information concerning a difficult term or word, try to use mental substitutes that are easier to understand.

The Trap of Familiarity

Don't just choose a word because you recognize it. On difficult questions, you may not recognize a number of words in the answer choices. The test writers don't put "make-believe" words on the test; so don't think that just because you only recognize all the words in one answer choice means that answer choice must be correct. If you only recognize words in one answer choice, then focus on that one. Is it correct? Try your best to determine if it is correct. If it is, that is great, but if it doesn't, eliminate it. Each word and answer choice you eliminate increases your chances of getting the question correct, even if you then have to guess among the unfamiliar choices.

Eliminate Answers

Eliminate choices as soon as you realize they are wrong. But be careful! Make sure you consider all of the possible answer choices. Just because one appears right, doesn't mean that the next one won't be even better! The test writers will usually put more than one good answer choice for every question, so read all of them. Don't worry if you are stuck between two that seem right. By getting down to just two remaining possible choices, your odds are now 50/50. Rather than wasting too much time, play the odds. You are guessing, but guessing wisely, because you've been able to knock out some of the answer choices that you know are wrong. If you are eliminating choices and realize that the last answer choice you are left with is also obviously wrong, don't panic. Start over and consider each choice again. There may easily be something that you missed the first time and will realize on the second pass.

Tough Questions

If you are stumped on a problem or it appears too hard or too difficult, don't waste time. Move on! Remember though, if you can quickly check for obviously incorrect answer choices, your chances of guessing correctly are greatly improved. Before you completely give up, at least try to knock out a couple of possible answers. Eliminate what you can and then guess at the remaining answer choices before moving on.

Brainstorm

If you get stuck on a difficult question, spend a few seconds quickly brainstorming. Run through the complete list of possible answer choices. Look at each choice and ask yourself, "Could this answer the question satisfactorily?" Go through each answer choice and consider it independently of the other. By systematically going through all possibilities, you may find something that you would otherwise overlook. Remember that when you get stuck, it's important to try to keep moving.

Read Carefully

Understand the problem. Read the question and answer choices carefully. Don't miss the question because you misread the terms. You have plenty of time to read each question thoroughly and make sure you understand what is being asked. Yet a happy medium must be attained, so don't waste too much time. You must read carefully, but efficiently.

Face Value
When in doubt, use common sense. Always accept the situation in the problem at face value. Don't read too much into it. These problems will not require you to make huge leaps of logic. The test writers aren't trying to throw you off with a cheap trick. If you have to go beyond creativity and make a leap of logic in order to have an answer choice answer the question, then you should look at the other answer choices. Don't overcomplicate the problem by creating theoretical relationships or explanations that will warp time or space. These are normal problems rooted in reality. It's just that the applicable relationship or explanation may not be readily apparent and you have to figure things out. Use your common sense to interpret anything that isn't clear.

Prefixes
If you're having trouble with a word in the question or answer choices, try dissecting it. Take advantage of every clue that the word might include. Prefixes and suffixes can be a huge help. Usually they allow you to determine a basic meaning. Pre- means before, post- means after, pro - is positive, de- is negative. From these prefixes and suffixes, you can get an idea of the general meaning of the word and try to put it into context. Beware though of any traps. Just because con is the opposite of pro, doesn't necessarily mean congress is the opposite of progress!

Hedge Phrases
Watch out for critical "hedge" phrases, such as likely, may, can, will often, sometimes, often, almost, mostly, usually, generally, rarely, sometimes. Question writers insert these hedge phrases to cover every possibility. Often an answer choice will be wrong simply because it leaves no room for exception. Avoid answer choices that have definitive words like "exactly," and "always".

Switchback Words
Stay alert for "switchbacks". These are the words and phrases frequently used to alert you to shifts in thought. The most common switchback word is "but". Others include although, however, nevertheless, on the other hand, even though, while, in spite of, despite, regardless of.

New Information
Correct answer choices will rarely have completely new information included. Answer choices typically are straightforward reflections of the material asked about and will directly relate to the question. If a new piece of information is included in an answer choice that doesn't even seem to relate to the topic being asked about, then that answer choice is likely incorrect. All of the information needed to answer the question is usually provided for you, and so you should not have to make guesses that are unsupported or choose answer choices that require unknown information that cannot be reasoned on its own.

Time Management
On technical questions, don't get lost on the technical terms. Don't spend too much time on any one question. If you don't know what a term means, then since you don't have a dictionary, odds are you aren't going to get much further. You should immediately recognize terms as whether or not you know them. If you don't, work with the other clues that you have, the other answer choices and terms provided, but don't waste too much time trying to figure out a difficult term.

Contextual Clues
Look for contextual clues. An answer can be right but not correct. The contextual clues will help you find the answer that is most right and is correct. Understand the context in which a phrase or statement is made. This will help you make important distinctions.

Don't Panic

Panicking will not answer any questions for you. Therefore, it isn't helpful. When you first see the question, if your mind goes blank, take a deep breath. Force yourself to mechanically go through the steps of solving the problem and using the strategies you've learned.

Pace Yourself

Don't get clock fever. It's easy to be overwhelmed when you're looking at a page full of questions, your mind is full of random thoughts and feeling confused, and the clock is ticking down faster than you would like. Calm down and maintain the pace that you have set for yourself. As long as you are on track by monitoring your pace, you are guaranteed to have enough time for yourself. When you get to the last few minutes of the test, it may seem like you won't have enough time left, but if you only have as many questions as you should have left at that point, then you're right on track!

Answer Selection

The best way to pick an answer choice is to eliminate all of those that are wrong, until only one is left and confirm that is the correct answer. Sometimes though, an answer choice may immediately look right. Be careful! Take a second to make sure that the other choices are not equally obvious. Don't make a hasty mistake. There are only two times that you should stop before checking other answers. First is when you are positive that the answer choice you have selected is correct. Second is when time is almost out and you have to make a quick guess!

Check Your Work

Since you will probably not know every term listed and the answer to every question, it is important that you get credit for the ones that you do know. Don't miss any questions through careless mistakes. If at all possible, try to take a second to look back over your answer selection and make sure you've selected the correct answer choice and haven't made a costly careless mistake (such as marking an answer choice that you didn't mean to mark). This quick double check should more than pay for itself in caught mistakes for the time it costs.

Beware of Directly Quoted Answers

Sometimes an answer choice will repeat word for word a portion of the question or reference section. However, beware of such exact duplication – it may be a trap! More than likely, the correct choice will paraphrase or summarize a point, rather than being exactly the same wording.

Slang

Scientific sounding answers are better than slang ones. An answer choice that begins "To compare the outcomes..." is much more likely to be correct than one that begins "Because some people insisted..."

Extreme Statements

Avoid wild answers that throw out highly controversial ideas that are proclaimed as established fact. An answer choice that states the "process should be used in certain situations, if..." is much more likely to be correct than one that states the "process should be discontinued completely." The first is a calm rational statement and doesn't even make a definitive, uncompromising stance, using a hedge word "if" to provide wiggle room, whereas the second choice is a radical idea and far more extreme.

Answer Choice Families

When you have two or more answer choices that are direct opposites or parallels, one of them is usually the correct answer. For instance, if one answer choice states "x increases" and another answer choice states "x decreases" or "y increases," then those two or three answer choices are very similar in construction and fall into the same family of answer choices. A family of answer choices is when two or three answer choices are very similar in construction, and yet often have a directly opposite meaning. Usually the correct answer choice will be in that family of answer choices. The "odd man out" or answer choice that doesn't seem to fit the parallel construction of the other answer choices is more likely to be incorrect.